Global and regional estimates of violence against women:

prevalence and health effects of intimate partner violence and non-partner sexual violence

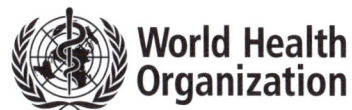
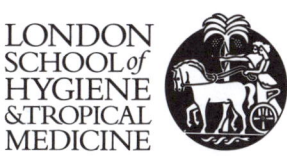
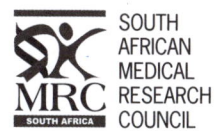

WHO Library Cataloguing-in-Publication Data:

Global and regional estimates of violence against women: prevalence and health effects of intimate partner violence and non-partner sexual violence.

1.Violence. 2.Spouse abuse. 3.Battered women – statistics and numerical data. 4.Sex offenses. 5.Women's health services. I.World Health Organization.

ISBN 978 92 4 156462 5 (NLM classification: HV 6625)

© World Health Organization 2013

All rights reserved. Publications of the World Health Organization are available on the WHO web site (www.who.int) or can be purchased from WHO Press, World Health Organization, 20 Avenue Appia, 1211 Geneva 27, Switzerland (tel.: +41 22 791 3264; fax: +41 22 791 4857; e-mail: bookorders@who.int).

Requests for permission to reproduce or translate WHO publications –whether for sale or for non-commercial distribution– should be addressed to WHO Press through the WHO web site (www.who.int/about/licensing/copyright_form/en/index.html).

The designations employed and the presentation of the material in this publication do not imply the expression of any opinion whatsoever on the part of the World Health Organization concerning the legal status of any country, territory, city or area or of its authorities, or concerning the delimitation of its frontiers or boundaries. Dotted lines on maps represent approximate border lines for which there may not yet be full agreement.

The mention of specific companies or of certain manufacturers' products does not imply that they are endorsed or recommended by the World Health Organization in preference to others of a similar nature that are not mentioned. Errors and omissions excepted, the names of proprietary products are distinguished by initial capital letters.

All reasonable precautions have been taken by the World Health Organization to verify the information contained in this publication. However, the published material is being distributed without warranty of any kind, either expressed or implied. The responsibility for the interpretation and use of the material lies with the reader. In no event shall the World Health Organization be liable for damages arising from its use.

Printed in Italy

Contents

Acknowledgements	**V**
Abbreviations	**VI**
Preface	**1**
Executive summary	**2**
Introduction	**4**
Definitions and conceptual framework	5
Health outcomes and causal pathways	5
Section 1: Methodology	**9**
Measurement of exposure to intimate partner violence and non-partner sexual violence	9
Definitions of WHO regions	9
Prevalence estimates of intimate partner violence	9
Compilation of evidence on the prevalence of intimate partner violence	10
Compilation of evidence on the prevalence of non-partner sexual violence	11
Methods to obtain regional and global prevalence estimates of intimate partner violence and non-partner sexual violence	13
Section 2: Results – lifetime prevalence estimates	**16**
Global and regional prevalence estimates of intimate partner violence	16
Global and regional prevalence estimates of non-partner sexual violence	18
Combined estimates of the prevalence of intimate partner violence and non-partner violence	20
Section 3: Results – the health effects of intimate partner violence and non-partner sexual violence	**21**
Health effects of exposure to intimate partner violence	21
HIV and other sexually transmitted infections	22
Induced abortion	23
Low birth weight and prematurity	23
Harmful alcohol use	24
Depression and suicide	24
Non-fatal injuries	25
Fatal injuries (intimate partner homicides)	26

Health effects of exposure to non-partner sexual violence	27
Depression and anxiety	27
Alcohol use disorders	28
Section 4: Summary and conclusions	**31**
Summary of findings	31
Limitations of the review	32
Implications of the findings	33
Research gaps	33
Conclusions	35
References	**37**
Appendix 1: Countries included by WHO region and age group	**44**
Appendix 2: Prevalence estimates of violence against women by Global Burden of Disease regions	**47**
Intimate partner violence	47
Non-partner sexual violence	48
Appendix 3: Regression models for calculating regional estimates of intimate partner violence and non-partner sexual violence	**49**
Regression function to estimate regional levels of intimate partner violence	49
Regression function to estimate age-group-specific regional levels of intimate partner violence	49
Regression function to estimate regional levels for non-partner sexual violence	50

Acknowledgements

This report was written by Claudia García-Moreno and Christina Pallitto of the Department of Reproductive Health and Research (RHR) of the World Health Organization (WHO), Karen Devries, Heidi Stöckl and Charlotte Watts of the London School of Hygiene and Tropical Medicine (LSHTM), and Naeemah Abrahams from the South African Medical Research Council (SAMRC). Max Petzold from the University of Gothenburg provided statistical support to all of the analyses.

The report is based on work done by the Expert Group on intimate partner violence, non- partner sexual violence and child sexual abuse for the Global Burden of Disease Study 2010, which was chaired by Charlotte Watts, LSHTM and Claudia García-Moreno, WHO. The systematic reviews of evidence on intimate partner violence were overseen by Karen Devries, LSHTM, and Christina Pallitto, WHO. The reviews of non-partner sexual violence were overseen by Naeemah Abrahams, SAMRC. Loraine Bacchus, Jennifer Child, Gail Falder, Amber Hill, Joelle Mak and Jennifer McCleary-Sills, also contributed to the systematic reviews.

Special thanks go to Gretchen Stevens and Colin Mathers of WHO's Department of Health Statistics and Information Systems, for their careful review of the data and methods for the estimations.

Thanks also to Michael Mbizvo and Marleen Temmerman, previous and current Director RHR for their support and inputs and to Catherine Hamill and Janette Petitpierre of RHR for the design and layout of the report.

The report was produced by RHR, WHO and edited by Penny Howes.

Abbreviations

AIDS	acquired immunodeficiency syndrome
aOR	adjusted odds ratio
CDC	Centers for Disease Control and Prevention
CES-D	Centre for Epidemiological Studies Depression Scale
CI	confidence interval
CINAHL	Cumulative Index to Nursing and Allied Health Literature
CTS	Conflict Tactics Scale
DHS	Demographic and Health Survey
DSM-IV	*Diagnostic and statistical manual of mental disorders*, fourth edition
GBD	Global Burden of Disease
GENACIS	*Gender, alcohol and culture: an international study*
HIV	human immunodeficiency virus
IMEMR	Index Medicus for the WHO Eastern Mediterranean Region
IMSEAR	Index Medicus for the WHO South-East Asia Region
IVAWS	International Violence Against Women Survey
LSHTM	London School of Hygiene and Tropical Medicine
OR	odds ratio
PTSD	post-traumatic stress disorder
RHS	reproductive health survey (CDC)
SAMRC	South African Medical Research Council
STI	sexually transmitted infection
USA	United States of America
WHO	World Health Organization
WPRIM	Western Pacific Region Index Medicus

Preface

Violence against women is not a new phenomenon, nor are its consequences to women's physical, mental and reproductive health. What is new is the growing recognition that acts of violence against women are not isolated events but rather form a pattern of behaviour that violates the rights of women and girls, limits their participation in society, and damages their health and well-being. When studied systematically, as was done with this report, it becomes clear that violence against women is a global public health problem that affects approximately one third of women globally.

By compiling and analysing all available data from studies designed to capture women's experiences of different forms of violence, this report provides the first such summary of the violent life events that many women experience. It documents not only how widespread this problem is, but also how deeply women's health is affected when they experience violence.

This report marks a big advance for women's health and rights. It adds to the momentum of the 57th session of the Commission on the Status of Women, which emphasized the need to address the root causes of violence against women and to strengthen multisectoral responses for women who have experienced violence. It also contributes to advocacy efforts such as the United Nations Secretary General's campaign UNiTE to end violence against women.

Action is clearly needed, and the health sector has an especially important role to play, considering the serious health risks faced by women and their families. WHO's new clinical and policy guidelines on the health sector response to violence against women provide specific evidence-based guidance that can help to strengthen the way health-care providers respond to women who have experienced violence. They also stress the importance of incorporating issues of violence into clinical training curricula, strengthening health systems to support women through direct services and multisectoral responses, identifying key entry points, such as sexual and reproductive health services and mental health services for addressing violence, and scaling up appropriate post-rape care responses.

No public health response is complete without prevention. Violence against women can and should be prevented. Promising programmes exist and many hinge on promoting gender equality so that the full potential of the world's women and girls can be realized. Let this report serve as a unified call to action for those working for a world without violence against women.

Flavia Bustreo
Assistant Director General
Family, Women and Children's Health
World Health Organization

Peter Piot
Director and Professor of Global Health,
London School of Hygiene & Tropical Medicine

Professor Salim S. Abdool Karim
President: South African Medical
Research Council

Oleg Chestnov
Assistant Director General
Noncommunicable Diseases and Mental Health
World Health Organization

Executive summary

"There is one universal truth, applicable to all countries, cultures and communities: violence against women is never acceptable, never excusable, never tolerable."

United Nations Secretary-General, Ban Ki-Moon (2008)[1]

Violence against women is a significant public health problem, as well as a fundamental violation of women's human rights.

This report, developed by the World Health Organization, the London School of Hygiene and Tropical Medicine and the South African Medical Research Council presents the first global systematic review and synthesis of the body of scientific data on the prevalence of two forms of violence against women — violence by an intimate partner (intimate partner violence) and sexual violence by someone other than a partner (non-partner sexual violence). It shows, for the first time, aggregated global and regional prevalence estimates of these two forms of violence, generated using population data from all over the world that have been compiled in a systematic way. The report also details the effects of violence on women's physical, sexual and reproductive, and mental health.

The findings are striking:

- overall, 35% of women worldwide have experienced either physical and/or sexual intimate partner violence or non-partner sexual violence. While there are many other forms of violence that women may be exposed to, this already represents a large proportion of the world's women;

- most of this violence is intimate partner violence. Worldwide, almost one third (30%) of all women who have been in a relationship have experienced physical and/or sexual violence by their intimate partner. In some regions, 38% of women have experienced intimate partner violence;

- globally, as many as 38% of all murders of women are committed by intimate partners;

- women who have been physically or sexually abused by their partners report higher rates of a number of important health problems. For example, they are 16% more likely to have a low-birth-weight baby. They are more than twice as likely to have an abortion, almost twice as likely to experience depression, and, in some regions, are 1.5 times more likely to acquire HIV, as compared to women who have not experienced partner violence;

- globally, 7% of women have been sexually assaulted by someone other than a partner. There are fewer data available on the health effects of non-partner sexual violence. However, the evidence that does exist reveals that women who have experienced this form of violence are 2.3 times more likely to have alcohol use disorders and 2.6 times more likely to experience depression or anxiety.

There is a clear need to scale up efforts across a range of sectors, both to prevent violence from happening in the first place and to provide necessary services for women experiencing violence.

---

1. *Secretary-General says violence against women never acceptable, never excusable, never tolerable, as he launches global campaign on issue.* New York, United Nations Department of Public Information, News and Media Division, 2008 (SG/SM/11437 WOM/1665).

The variation in the prevalence of violence seen within and between communities, countries and regions, highlights that violence is not inevitable, and that it can be prevented. Promising prevention programmes exist, and need to be tested and scaled up.[2] There is growing evidence about what factors explain the global variation documented. This evidence highlights the need to address the economic and sociocultural factors that foster a culture of violence against women. This also includes the importance of challenging social norms that support male authority and control over women and sanction or condone violence against women; reducing levels of childhood exposures to violence; reforming discriminatory family law; strengthening women's economic and legal rights; and eliminating gender inequalities in access to formal wage employment and secondary education.

Services also need to be provided for those who have experienced violence. The health sector must play a greater role in responding to intimate partner violence and sexual violence against women. WHO's new clinical and policy guidelines on the health-sector response to violence against women emphasize the urgent need to integrate issues related to violence into clinical training. It is important that all health-care providers understand the relationship between exposure to violence and women's ill health, and are able to respond appropriately. One key aspect is to identify opportunities to provide support and link women with other services they need – for example, when women seek sexual and reproductive health services (e.g. antenatal care, family planning, post-abortion care) or HIV testing, mental health and emergency services. Comprehensive post-rape care services need to be made available and accessible at a much larger scale than is currently provided.

The report shows that violence against women is pervasive globally. The findings send a powerful message that violence against women is not a small problem that only occurs in some pockets of society, but rather is a global public health problem of epidemic proportions, requiring urgent action. It is time for the world to take action: a life free of violence is a basic human right, one that every woman, man and child deserves.

---

2. Preventing intimate partner violence and sexual violence against women. Taking action and generating evidence. Geneva, World Health Organization, 2010.

Introduction

There is growing recognition that violence against women has a large public health impact, in addition to being a gross violation of women's human rights (*1*). This recognition is the result of international commitments to document the magnitude of the problem and its consequences and the ever-expanding evidence base on the prevalence and consequences of this violence. The United Nations Secretary-General, Ban Ki-Moon, has issued a global call to action to end violence against women, by launching the UNiTE to End Violence against Women campaign. Most recently, the agreed conclusions of the 57th session of the Commission on the Status of Women (*2*) emphasize the importance both of addressing structural and underlying causes and risk factors in order to prevent violence against women and girls, and of strengthening multisectoral services, programmes and responses for victims and survivors. The agreed conclusions also call for continued multidisciplinary research and analysis on the causes of, and cost and risk factors for, violence against women and girls, in order to inform laws, policies and strategies and support awareness-raising efforts.

The term "violence against women" encompasses many forms of violence, including violence by an intimate partner (intimate partner violence) and rape/sexual assault and other forms of sexual violence perpetrated by someone other than a partner (non-partner sexual violence), as well as female genital mutilation, honour killings and the trafficking of women.

This report focuses on two forms of violence against women: physical and/or sexual intimate partner violence and non-partner sexual violence. Over the past decade, there has been a rapid growth in the body of research evidence available on the prevalence of intimate partner violence and its health effects. This is, in part, a result of a growing consensus on how best to measure women's exposure to intimate partner (and other forms of) violence through household surveys, while also taking precautions to put women's safety first and to ensure that respondents requesting assistance can be referred to services if needed (*3*). As well as specialized surveys, national governments are increasingly incorporating questions on women's exposure to partner violence into their national health surveys, including, for example, in the Demographic and Health Surveys (DHSs) (*4*) and the Centers for Disease Control and Prevention (CDC) reproductive health surveys (RHSs) (*5*).

Similarly, for sexual violence by perpetrators other than a partner (i.e., friends, acquaintances, strangers, other family members), there is a growing body of research evidence on levels of such violence, although this is much more limited than for intimate partner violence. There is growing consensus on how best to document exposure to sexual violence, although, in practice, definitions may vary between studies, and not all forms of sexual violence are well documented.

This report presents the first global systematic review and synthesis of the body of scientific data measuring the population prevalence of intimate partner violence against women, and non-partner sexual violence against women. It presents, for the first time, aggregated global and regional prevalence estimates of these two forms of violence, generated using population data from all over the world, compiled in a systematic way.

The report is divided into three sections, with a fourth summary and conclusions section. Section 1 describes the methods used for calculating the global and regional prevalence estimates of intimate partner violence and non-partner sexual violence,[3] and section 2 presents the global and regional prevalence estimates for each form of violence. Section 3 summarizes evidence on the magnitude of a range of health effects associated with exposure to either form of violence. These analyses are based on systematic reviews and data pooled across surveys, analysed using meta-analysis where possible. This evidence shows that women experiencing intimate partner violence are significantly more likely to experience serious health problems than women who have not experienced such violence. The health effects of non-partner sexual violence are also presented, although fewer outcomes are included in this section because of the relative lack of research in this area.

This evidence shows that both intimate partner violence and non-partner sexual violence are widespread and that they have important effects on women's physical, sexual and reproductive, and mental health. In combination, these findings send a powerful message that violence against women is not a small problem that only occurs in some pockets of society, but rather is a global public health problem of epidemic proportions, requiring urgent action.

Definitions and conceptual framework

Table 1 summarizes the working definitions for each form of violence used in this review.

Health outcomes and causal pathways

While there has been an important growth during the past decade in the number of population-based studies globally that are starting to document the prevalence/magnitude of different forms of violence against women, there has been less research on the health effects of exposures to different forms of violence (6). However, what this literature does highlight is the extreme breadth in potential health effects – encompassing physical, sexual and reproductive, and mental health, with potentially large impacts on levels of women's morbidity and mortality. This evidence comes from a few rigorous, prospective and carefully controlled clinical and epidemiological research studies, and, more commonly, from assessments of association using population-based cross-sectional data. As described in more detail below, although the field's reliance on cross-sectional data is a limitation, the studies used are often large, representative, population-based surveys that have been replicated in multiple settings, with strong consistency of findings across studies.

The likely causal pathways between different forms of exposure to violence and different health outcomes are starting to be documented and understood better. These pathways are often complex, with context-specific, physiological, behavioural and other factors influencing the likelihood of disease/ill-health outcomes.

There is a broad range of health effects. Figure 1 shows the hypothesized pathways through which intimate partner violence leads to different forms of morbidity and mortality. These include the direct pathway of violence resulting in injury and death, and the other direct and indirect pathways for multiple health problems for women, as well as maternal and perinatal health outcomes.

---

3. The age of 15 years is set as the lower age limit for partner violence and non-partner sexual violence, so while we refer to "violence against women" throughout the report, we recognize that violence experienced by girls between the ages of 15 and 18 years is also considered child maltreatment.

Table 1. Working definitions of forms of exposure to violence used in this review

Term	Definition for this review
Intimate partner violence[a]	Self-reported experience of one or more acts of physical and/or sexual violence by a current or former partner since the age of 15 years.[b] • Physical violence is defined as: being slapped or having something thrown at you that could hurt you, being pushed or shoved, being hit with a fist or something else that could hurt, being kicked, dragged or beaten up, being choked or burnt on purpose, and/or being threatened with, or actually, having a gun, knife or other weapon used on you. • Sexual violence is defined as: being physically forced to have sexual intercourse when you did not want to, having sexual intercourse because you were afraid of what your partner might do, and/or being forced to do something sexual that you found humiliating or degrading.[c]
Severe intimate partner violence	Is defined on the basis of the severity of the acts of physical violence: being beaten up, choked or burnt on purpose, and/or being threatened or having a weapon used against you is considered severe. Any sexual violence is also considered severe.
Current intimate partner violence	Self-reported experience of partner violence in the past year.
Prior intimate partner violence	Self-reported experience of partner violence before the past year.
Non-partner sexual violence	When aged 15 years or over,[b] experience of being forced to perform any sexual act that you did not want to by someone other than your husband/partner.

[a] The definition of intimate partner varies between settings and includes formal partnerships, such as marriage, as well as informal partnerships, including dating relationships and unmarried sexual relationships. In some settings, intimate partners tend to be married, while in others more informal partnerships are more common.

[b] The age of 15 years is set as the lower age range for partner violence and non-partner sexual violence. Intimate partner violence has only been measured for women who have reported being in a partnership, as they are the "at-risk" group. Therefore, for women between the ages of 15 and 18 years, only those who have been in a partnership, including dating relationships and marital relationships in settings where marriage occurs in this age group, could potentially report intimate partner violence. Young women in the age group 15–18 years experiencing non-partner sexual violence can also be considered, by some legal definitions, to have experienced child sexual abuse, as these are not mutually exclusive categories.

[c] The definition of humiliating and degrading may vary across studies, depending on the regional and cultural setting.

A more indirect pathway, mediated by stress responses, is documented in a body of research that has expanded rapidly over the past two decades. This literature provides good evidence about the underlying biological (physiological) mechanisms of the association between exposures to violence and different adverse health outcomes, through complex and interconnected neural, neuroendocrine and immune responses to acute and chronic stress (7–9). For example, when exposed to prolonged or acute stress, areas of the brain such as the hippocampus, amygdala and prefrontal cortex undergo structural changes that have implications for mental health and cognitive functioning, and can lead to mental disorders, somatoform disorders or chronic illness, as well as other physical conditions (10). In response to stress, the immune system can be compromised, exacerbating the spread of cancer and viral infections. Sustained and acute elevated stress levels have also been linked to cardiovascular disease, hypertension, gastrointestinal disorders, chronic pain, and the development of insulin-dependent diabetes (10). Stress during and around the time of pregnancy has been linked with low-birth-weight infants, as rising cortisol levels lead to constriction of the blood vessels, limiting blood flow to the uterus. Furthermore, the hypothalamic–pituitary–adrenal response can trigger premature labour and premature birth, through contractions of the smooth muscle tissue in the uterus (11, 12).

In addition to the biological stress response, there are behavioural and other risk factors that also influence the link between intimate partner violence and adverse health outcomes. Some women try to manage the negative consequences of abuse through the use of alcohol, prescription medication, tobacco or other drugs (13, 14). Each of these is an important risk factor for poor health, and part of the complex link between exposures to violence and other health risk factors that mediate negative health outcomes.

An additional, less documented, but emerging pathway relates to the psychological control that defines many relationships in which partner violence occurs. These controlling behaviours relate to a series of ways in which male partners might attempt to control and/or limit the behaviours and social interactions of their female partners (e.g., limiting social and family interactions, insisting on knowing where she is at all times, being suspicious of unfaithfulness, getting angry if she speaks with another man, expecting his permission for seeking health care). Such controlling behaviour often co-occurs with physical and sexual violence, and may be highly prevalent in violent relationships. Emerging evidence suggests that abusive partners who exhibit these behaviours can limit women's ability to control their sexual and reproductive decision-making, their access to health care, or their adherence to medications, which can have adverse health effects.

As illustrated in Figure 1, the relationship between exposures to violence and health effects is complex. Intrinsic in many of these postulated associations is the assumption that there are intermediate pathways, such that violence might increase the tendency to a particular risk behaviour and that risk behaviour, in turn, increases the likelihood of an adverse health outcome. The data to date, however, are limited; they are mostly cross-sectional and do not allow temporality or causality to be determined. More and different kinds of research, such as longitudinal studies, inclusion of biomarkers to measure health outcomes, and properly controlling for potentially confounding variables affecting the associations found, are needed to be able to describe these pathways and associations more conclusively.

Figure 1. Pathways and health effects on intimate partner violence

```
                        INTIMATE PARTNER VIOLENCE
                ┌───────────────┬───────────────────┐
                ▼               ▼                   ▼
        PHYSICAL TRAUMA   PSYCHOLOGICAL        FEAR AND CONTROL
                           TRAUMA/STRESS
```

- **INJURY**
  - musculoskeletal
  - soft tissue
  - genital trauma
  - other

- **MENTAL HEALTH PROBLEMS**
  - PTSD
  - anxiety
  - depression
  - eating disorders
  - suicidality

- **LIMITED SEXUAL AND REPRODUCTIVE CONTROL**
  - lack of contraception
  - unsafe sex

- **HEALTH CARE SEEKING**
  - lack of autonomy
  - difficulties seeking care and other services

- **SUBSTANCE USE**
  - alcohol
  - other drugs
  - tobacco

- **NONCOMMUNICABLE DISEASES**
  - cardiovascular disease
  - hypertension

- **SOMATOFORM**
  - irritable bowel
  - chronic pain
  - chronic pelvic pain

- **PERINATAL/MATERNAL HEALTH**
  - low birth weight
  - prematurity
  - pregnancy loss

- **SEXUAL AND REPRODUCTIVE HEALTH**
  - unwanted pregnancy
  - abortion
  - HIV
  - other STIs
  - gynaecological problems

DISABILITY

DEATH
- homicide • suicide • other

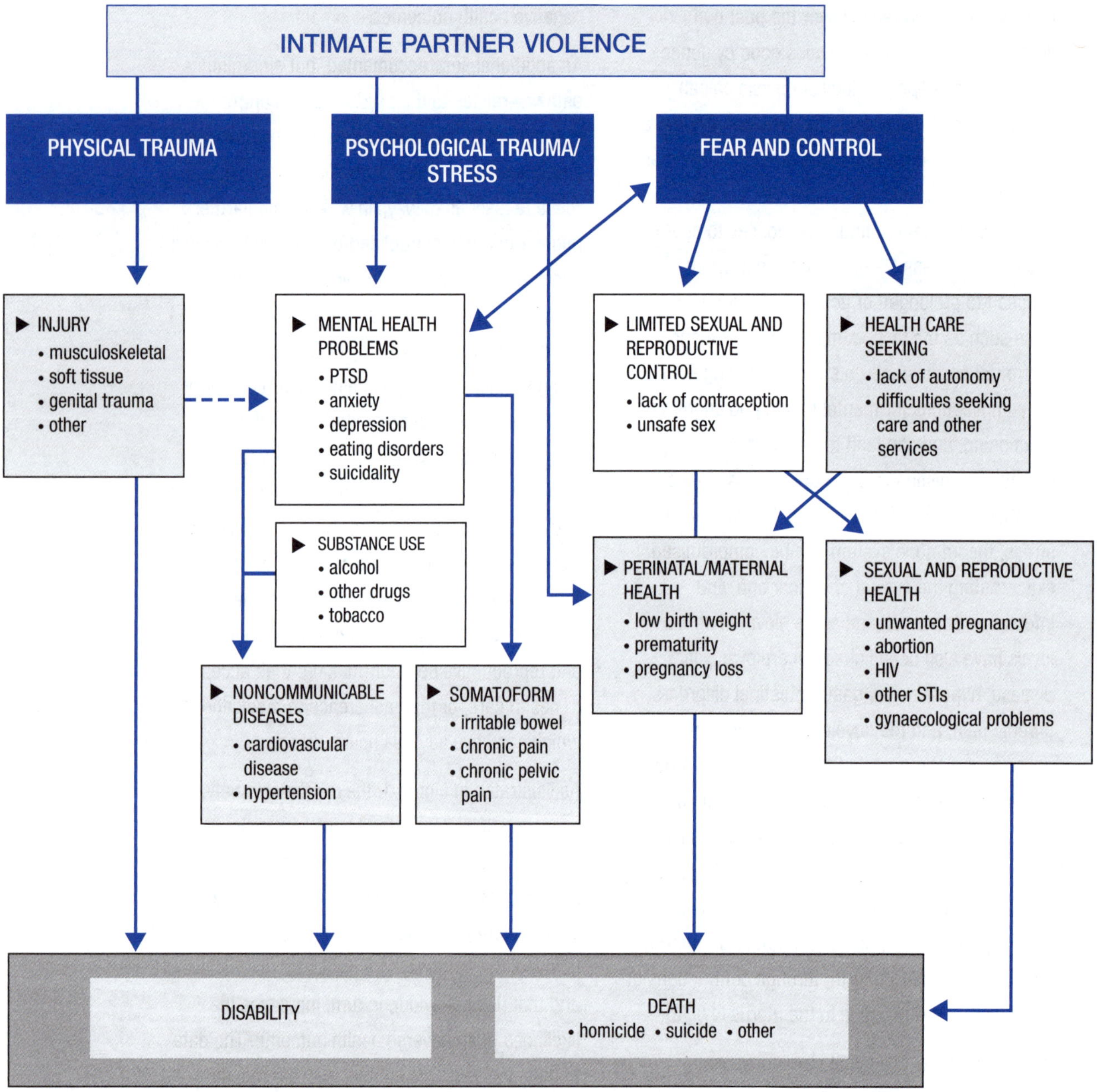

There are multiple pathways through which intimate partner violence can lead to adverse health outcomes. This figure highlights three key mechanisms and pathways that can explain many of these outcomes. Mental health problems and substance use might result directly from any of the three mechanisms, which might, in turn, increase health risks. However, mental health problems and substance use are not necessarily a precondition for subsequent health effects, and will not always lie in the pathway to adverse health.

Section 1: Methodology

This section of the report briefly describes the methods used for calculating the global and regional prevalence estimates of intimate partner violence and non-partner sexual violence.

Measurement of exposure to intimate partner violence and non-partner sexual violence

There is growing consensus on how to measure exposures to different forms of interpersonal violence, with most work focusing on the measurement of violence by an intimate partner (15, 16). Gold standard methods to estimate the prevalence of any form of violence are obtained by asking respondents direct questions about their experience of specific acts of violence over a defined period of time, rather than using more generic questions about whether the respondent has been "abused" or has experienced "domestic violence" or "rape" or "sexual abuse", which tends to yield less disclosure. Methodological issues related to the implementation of the survey procedures – including the selection and levels of training of interviewers, and ensuring appropriate support of respondents and interviewers, have also been shown to influence levels of disclosure (3, 17, 18).

Definitions of WHO regions

The focus of this review was to obtain both global and regional evidence on the prevalence of intimate partner violence and non-partner sexual violence. The regional assessments in this report were based upon the World Health Organization (WHO) regions, and included low- and middle-income countries in the Region of the Americas (Latin America and the Caribbean), the African Region, the Eastern Mediterranean Region, the European Region, the South-East Asia Region, and the Western Pacific Region, as well as a category for high-income countries from the different regions (See Appendix 1 for tables detailing the countries for which data are available in each region).

The global estimate for intimate partner violence and non-partner sexual violence is based on the regional weighted prevalence estimates using Global Burden of Disease (GBD) regions (19), since these regions are broken into finer categories that are more meaningful epidemiologically. Regional estimates for intimate partner violence and non-partner sexual violence for these regions are included in Tables A2.1 and A2.2 in Appendix 2.

Prevalence estimates of intimate partner violence

Most population-based research to assess the prevalence of intimate partner violence focuses on compiling information on respondents' exposures to a range of physical, sexual and emotional/psychological acts of violence by a current or former intimate partner, whether cohabiting or not. Definitions of each of these aspects of violence are operationalized using behaviourally specific questions related to each type of violence, ranging from slaps, pushes and shoves, through to more severe acts, such as being strangled or burnt, hit with a fist, threatened with, or having, a weapon used against you. The Conflict Tactics Scale (CTS) (20) has been widely used in the United States of America (USA) and elsewhere to document the prevalence of physical partner violence, framing violent acts in the context of relationship conflict. The *WHO multi-country study on women's health and domestic violence against women* (21) and the violence against women module of the DHS (22) are adapted versions of the CTS that also ask about a set of behaviourally specific acts that women experience, without framing the questions as gradations of relationship conflict, but rather as independent acts in a constellation of experiences encompassing partner violence. These instruments have been applied in numerous settings and are considered valid and reliable measures of intimate partner violence.

In general, surveys on intimate partner violence ask respondents about their exposure ever (in their lifetime), and in the past year, with a few studies also asking about violence in the last month or within a particular relationship. This report focuses on assessing women's lifetime exposure to physical or sexual violence, or both, by an intimate partner. This is defined as the proportion of ever-partnered women who reported having experienced one or more acts of physical or sexual violence, or both, by a current or former intimate partner at any point in their lives (See Table 1, footnote *a* for a definition of intimate partner). Current prevalence is defined as the proportion of ever-partnered women reporting that at least one act of physical or sexual violence, or both, took place during the 12 months prior to the interview.

It should be noted that intimate partner violence also includes emotional abuse (being humiliated, insulted, intimidated or threatened, for example) and controlling behaviours by a partner, such as not being allowed to see friends or family (*23, 24*). This form of abuse also impacts the health of individuals. However, there is currently a lack of agreement on standard measures of emotional/psychological partner violence and the threshold at which acts that can be considered unkind or insulting cross the line into being emotional abuse. For this reason, emotional/psychological violence has not been included in this analysis, and, for the purposes of this report, the measures of intimate partner violence solely include act(s) of physical and/or sexual violence.

Compilation of evidence on the prevalence of intimate partner violence

A systematic review of the prevalence of intimate partner violence was conducted, compiling evidence from both peer-reviewed literature and grey literature from first record to 2008; the peer-reviewed component was then updated to 9 January 2011. For this, a search was conducted of 26 medical and social science databases in all languages, yielding results in English, Spanish, French, Portuguese, Russian, Chinese and a few other languages. Controlled vocabulary terms specific to each database were used (e.g. MeSH terms for Medline). Only representative population-based studies with prevalence estimates for intimate partner violence in women of any age above 15 years were included. Any author definitions of intimate partner violence were included. A total of 7350 abstracts were screened. Additional analysis of the *WHO multi-country study on women's health and domestic violence against women* (*21*) (10 countries) was also performed, and additional analyses of the International Violence Against Women Surveys (IVAWS, 8 countries) (*25*), *GENACIS: Gender, alcohol and culture: an international study* (16 countries) (*26*) and the DHS (20 countries) (*4, 22*) were also conducted. In total, 185 studies from 86 countries representing all global regions met our inclusion criteria, and data from 155 studies in 81 countries informed our estimates. Of these, 141 studies were used in the all ages model, 89 were used in the age-specific model, and 75 were used in both. Of the 14 studies used only in the age-specific model, nine had insufficient data for calculating an all-age estimate and five had a broader range of age specific data but were not included in the all-age estimate.

Sixty-six studies had prevalence data for a broad age band so were included in the all ages model but not in the age-specific model.

The study focused on extracting data by age group on ever, and past-year, experience of physical and sexual violence for ever-partnered women, making note of the specific definitions used, as well as elements of the survey characteristics. Where a breakdown by the severity of violence was reported, these data were also compiled. For this, severe violence was categorized by the severity of the acts of physical violence, so that any severe acts experienced, such as being beaten up, choked or burnt on purpose, threatened with a weapon, or a woman having had a weapon used against her, as well as any act of sexual violence, would be considered severe violence.

Only studies with primary data from population surveys were included, and only women aged 15 years and older were included. In some settings, girls are partnered formally or informally before the age of 15 years, but since most surveys capturing data on intimate partner violence, especially those from low- and middle-income countries, focus on women in the reproductive age group (15–49 years), 15 years was set as the lower age limit for data extraction. Intimate partner violence experienced by girls aged under 18 years can also be considered child abuse or maltreatment, and we stress the importance of recognizing that these are not mutually exclusive categories (See Table 1, footnote b).

Similarly, data on women aged over 49 years were scarce and tended to be from high-income countries. However, data were extracted for older age categories, where these had been collected. Tables A1.3 and A1.4 in Appendix 1 show the distribution of studies by age group and for all ages by region for data on intimate partner violence.

Intimate partner violence against older women is a form of elder maltreatment, and, as is the case with child maltreatment, the categories of intimate partner violence and elder maltreatment are not mutually exclusive. Violence against children and the elderly are important areas of research that merit further investigation and careful consideration of the special methodological and safety concerns inherent in research among these populations.

Compilation of evidence on the prevalence of non-partner sexual violence

A systematic search was used to compile evidence on the prevalence of non-partner sexual violence. For this, a systematic search of biomedical databases was carried out (*British Medical Journal*, British Nursing Index, Cumulative Index to Nursing and Allied Health Literature [CINAHL], Cochrane Library, Embase, Health Management Information Consortium, Medline, PubMed, Science Direct, Wiley-Interscience), as well as social sciences databases (International Bibliography of Social Sciences, PsychINFO, Web of Science) and international databases (ADOLEC, African Healthline, Global Health, Index Medicus for the WHO Eastern Mediterranean Region (IMEMR), Index Medicus for the South-East Asian Region (IMSEAR) and the Western Pacific Region Index Medicus (WPRIM), LILACS, Medcarib, Popline) for studies published from 1998 to 2010. An independent search was also conducted of international surveys on violence against women or surveys that included questions on exposure to non-partner sexual violence. Specific data sets included: IVAWS (25); the *WHO multi-country study on women's health and domestic violence against women* (*21*); DHS (*4, 22*); GENACIS (*26*); CDC RHS (*5*) and crime surveys across the globe. Citations were also followed up and contact was made with experts, giving special attention to studies from conflict settings, to identify additional studies.

Studies with primary data on population-based estimates of non-partner sexual violence were included and non-population-based studies were only considered in regions where population data were limited. Only women aged 15 years and older were included, to differentiate violence against women from child sexual abuse and to be consistent with the estimates of intimate partner violence. We again acknowledge, however, that sexual violence occurring between the ages of 15 and 18 years is also considered child sexual abuse and that these categories are not mutually exclusive.

Data on lifetime and current (past year) exposure to non-partner sexual violence were extracted, but it was generally found that current exposure to non-partner sexual violence was reported rarely. The way in which perpetrators were defined in studies was critical in assessing inclusion. For exposure, sexual violence by all perpetrators other than intimate partners (e.g., strangers, acquaintances, friends, family members, colleagues, police, military personnel, etc.) was relevant to the analysis. Many studies combined perpetrators (intimate partners and non-partner perpetrators) in the analysis, and studies where intimate partner perpetrators could not be separated from non-partners were excluded in order to avoid double counting of acts captured in the analysis of intimate partner violence. For example, many crime surveys (European Survey of Crime and Safety) (27) and International Crime Victim Survey (28) presented data on sexual victimization, without differentiating perpetrators.

Some studies only reported on single perpetrators, such as strangers, while many combined non-partner perpetrators. To prevent double counting and overlapping of estimates from studies where estimates were provided for multiple single perpetrators (stranger, acquaintance, family member), the estimate based on the largest sample was chosen.

Estimates based on any author's definition of sexual violence were included. Unlike intimate partner violence, most studies used a single broad question such as "Have you ever been forced to have sex or to perform a sexual act when you did not want to with someone other than your partner?", which is known to underestimate prevalence. To prevent double counting, estimates from the same study/author were checked and the most relevant paper/estimates were included.

The majority of the study estimates (87%) were derived from three large international data sets: the *WHO multi-country study on women's health and domestic violence against women* (21) (10 countries), IVAWS (25) (8 countries) and GENACIS (26) (16 countries). All three studies used a single question to capture exposure to non-partner sexual violence since the age of 15 years. All the available DHSs were reviewed (4) and since only eight of the 48 surveys provided data on sexual violence by non-partners, only these eight surveys could be included.

Sexual violence during conflict perpetrated by militia, military personnel or police is an important aspect of non-partner sexual violence. Only six population studies were identified that reported on non-partner sexual violence in conflict-affected settings. Many other studies report on sexual violence, as described in a recent review – but few of them are population-based studies or they do not separate partner and non-partner sexual violence (29). In this review, two of the studies in conflict settings were part of larger multi-country studies: the Philippines was part of the IVAWS (25) and Sri Lanka was part of the GENACIS project

(*26*), while the others (*29–34*) were studies dedicated to measuring experiences of violence during conflict.

A total of 7231 abstracts/records were identified for screening and the main reasons for exclusion were incorrect study design/non-population studies and studies focused on intimate partner violence or combining perpetrators. A total of 189 records/abstracts were identified for full-text screening and, after assessment, 77 studies covering 56 countries were included, producing 412 estimates from 347 605 participating women aged 15 years and older. Data were found for five of the six WHO regions, with no data identified for the WHO Eastern Mediterranean Region. Table A1.2 in Appendix 1 shows a list of the 56 countries and territories for which data were available.

During data extraction, prevalence estimates were compiled by age group, and data on key methodological issues related to the context of the study (such as in a conflict setting), or study methods (including the question used to ask about sexual violence) were included. In practice, more than half (59.7%) of the estimates were derived from dedicated studies on violence against women, and 83.7% were from the three major multi-country studies (WHO, IVAWS, GENACIS). The majority of estimates measured lifetime non-partner sexual violence (81.8%), combined non-partner perpetrators of sexual violence (93.7%), and used a broad definition of sexual violence (91.5%).

Methods to obtain regional and global prevalence estimates of intimate partner violence and non-partner sexual violence

Using estimates from all of these data sources, separately for both intimate partner violence and non-partner sexual violence, a random effects meta-regression (the metareg command version sbe23_1 using residual maximum likelihood with a Knapp–Hartung modification to the variance of the estimated coefficients, Stata 12.1) (*35, 36*) was fitted to produce adjusted prevalence estimates for all WHO regions and by age groups (only for intimate partner violence) (*37*). The estimates of intimate partner violence were adjusted for differences in definitions of violence (physical or sexual or both), time periods of measurement (lifetime versus current), severity of violence (whether moderate or severe), and whether a study was national or subnational (national models being more generalizable) (see Appendix 3 for model descriptions). The covariates adjusted for in the model for non-partner sexual violence included whether fieldworkers were trained (interviewers specially trained in violence research tend to elicit more reliable responses from respondents as opposed to those who do not receive the specialized training), whether the study was a national study (and therefore more generalizable to the population of the country as a whole), and whether the respondent was given a choice of multiple perpetrators as opposed to a single perpetrator (multiple response options yield more accurate disclosure). More details on the methodology are provided in two forthcoming papers on the prevalence of intimate partner violence and non-partner sexual violence respectively (*37, 38*).

WHO region was included in the model as a dummy variable, producing adjusted regional estimates (See Appendix 1 for countries included in each of the WHO regions for which data were available). In a second step of the analysis, using regional estimates derived from regression models developed for the Global Burden of Disease regions (See Appendix 2.1), as described elsewhere (37), the global estimate was calculated by weighting the GBD regional estimates together, based on the United Nations statistics for the total population of women aged 15–49 years for each region in 2010 (39). The GBD regions, as opposed to the WHO regions, were used to calculate the global prevalence, because the high-income category of the WHO regions comprised countries from multiple geographic regions, which affected the population weighting for the remaining countries in each of the WHO regions and resulted in a weighted global prevalence estimate that differed very slightly (by less than 1%) from the global prevalence derived from the GBD regions.

For intimate partner violence, only studies of ever-partnered women were included. The estimates were then adjusted such that they reflected the proportion of the total population of women experiencing intimate partner violence, by multiplying the estimates by the age and study year and the country-specific proportion of women who had ever had sexual intercourse, which was assumed to be a proxy for "ever-partnered" (personal communication, S Lim, Associate Professor of Global Health, Institute for Health Metrics and Evaluation at the University of Washington, 2013).

For intimate partner violence, only the studies reporting estimates for "all ages" were included in the regional prevalence estimates, while for non-partner sexual violence, age-specific estimates were also included if no data for "all ages" were reported for the particular study.

Age-group-specific prevalence rates were estimated for intimate partner violence, but not for non-partner sexual violence, owing to the limited number of studies with prevalence estimates by age for non-partner sexual violence. Included age-group-specific estimates were categorized into the following age groups: 15–19, 20–24, 25–34, 35–44, 45–54, 55–64, 65–74, 75–84 and 85+ years. To obtain the global age group specific estimates the regional estimates were weighted together based on the regional female population size for the year 2010 (37, 38). Region-specific age-group estimates were produced by combining the dummy variable for region and the dummy variable for age group, obtaining all unique combinations. Global age-group-specific estimates were finally obtained by weighting the regional age-group estimates by the total regional population of women in that age group. It should be noted that the age-specific estimates and the "all ages" estimate do not correspond to each other or to any region since age-specific estimates were calculated using studies reporting age-specific results, and results for "all ages" were calculated including only those studies explicitly reporting an estimate for "all ages".

An estimate of the combined proportion of physical and/or sexual intimate partner violence and non-partner sexual violence was calculated by using data from the regional prevalence results presented in this report for non-partner sexual violence and for the regional prevalence results of intimate partner violence among all women. The proportion of all women who had experienced physical or sexual intimate partner violence and/or non-partner sexual violence for each region was calculated using the following formula:

$$a*(100-c)+b$$

where a is the proportion of all women who had experienced intimate partner violence, from the prevalence estimates for all women (results presented in the report for intimate partner violence are among ever partnered women but for the combined estimate are for all women); b is the proportion of women who had experienced non-partner sexual violence, from the prevalence estimates; and c is the proportion of women who had experienced both intimate partner physical and sexual violence and non-partner sexual violence. The relative proportion of women who had experienced intimate partner violence and had also experienced non-partner sexual violence (c) was calculated using regional data from the original 10 countries (15 sites) participating in the *WHO multi-country study on women's health and domestic violence against women* (*21*), in which questions on both intimate partner violence and non-partner sexual violence were asked of the same women. Global estimates were calculated using population weights for the WHO regions, resulting in a global prevalence that shows the proportion of women who had experienced intimate partner violence or non-partner sexual violence, or both.

Section 2: Results – lifetime prevalence estimates

Global and regional prevalence estimates of intimate partner violence

This section presents the global and regional prevalence estimates of intimate partner violence and non-partner sexual violence. This is the first time that such a comprehensive compilation of all available global data has been used to obtain global and regional prevalence estimates. Estimates are based on data extracted from 79 countries and two territories.

The global prevalence of physical and/or sexual intimate partner violence among all ever-partnered women was 30.0% (95% confidence interval [CI] = 27.8% to 32.2%). The prevalence was highest in the WHO African, Eastern Mediterranean and South-East Asia Regions, where approximately 37% of ever-partnered women reported having experienced physical and/or sexual intimate partner violence at some point in their lives (see Table 2). Respondents in the Region of the Americas reported the next highest prevalence, with approximately 30% of women reporting lifetime exposure. Prevalence was lower in the high-income region (23%) and in the European and the Western Pacific Regions, where 25% of ever-partnered women reported lifetime intimate partner violence experience (see Figure 2).[4]

> The global lifetime prevalence of intimate partner violence among ever-partnered women is 30.0% (95% CI = 27.8% to 32.2%.)

Table 3 shows the lifetime prevalence of intimate partner violence by age groups among ever-partnered women. What is striking is that the prevalence of exposure to violence is already high among young women aged 15–19 years, suggesting that violence commonly starts early in women's relationships. Prevalence then progressively rises to reach its peak in the age group of 40–44 years. The reported prevalence among women aged 50 years and older is lower, although the confidence intervals around these estimates are quite large, and a closer examination of the data reveals that data for the older age groups come primarily from high-income countries (see Table A1.3 in Appendix 1). Since most of the surveys on violence against women or other surveys with a violence module, such as the DHS or RHS, are carried out on women aged 15 or 18 to 49 years, fewer data points are available for the over-49 age group. For this reason, it should not be interpreted that older women have experienced lower levels of partner violence, but rather that less is known about patterns of violence among women aged 50 years and older, especially in low- and middle-income countries.

---

4. More recent studies from the Western Pacific Region using the WHO study methodology have since been published, but were not available at the time the data were compiled. They show very high prevalence rates of physical and/or sexual intimate partner violence between 60% and 68% (40–42).

Table 2. Lifetime prevalence of physical and/or sexual intimate partner violence among ever-partnered women by WHO region

WHO region	Prevalence, %	95% CI, %
Low- and middle-income regions:		
Africa	36.6	32.7 to 40.5
Americas	29.8	25.8 to 33.9
Eastern Mediterranean	37.0	30.9 to 43.1
Europe	25.4	20.9 to 30.0
South-East Asia	37.7	32.8 to 42.6
Western Pacific	24.6	20.1 to 29.0
High income	23.2	20.2 to 26.2

CI = confidence interval.

Table 3. Lifetime prevalence of intimate partner violence by age group among ever-partnered women

Age group, years	Prevalence, %	95% CI, %
15–19	29.4	26.8 to 32.1
20–24	31.6	29.2 to 33.9
25–29	32.3	30.0 to 34.6
30–34	31.1	28.9 to 33.4
35–39	36.6	30.0 to 43.2
40–44	37.8	30.7 to 44.9
45–49	29.2	26.9 to 31.5
50–54	25.5	18.6 to 32.4
55–59	15.1	6.1 to 24.1
60–64	19.6	9.6 to 29.5
65–69	22.2	12.8 to 31.6

CI = confidence interval.

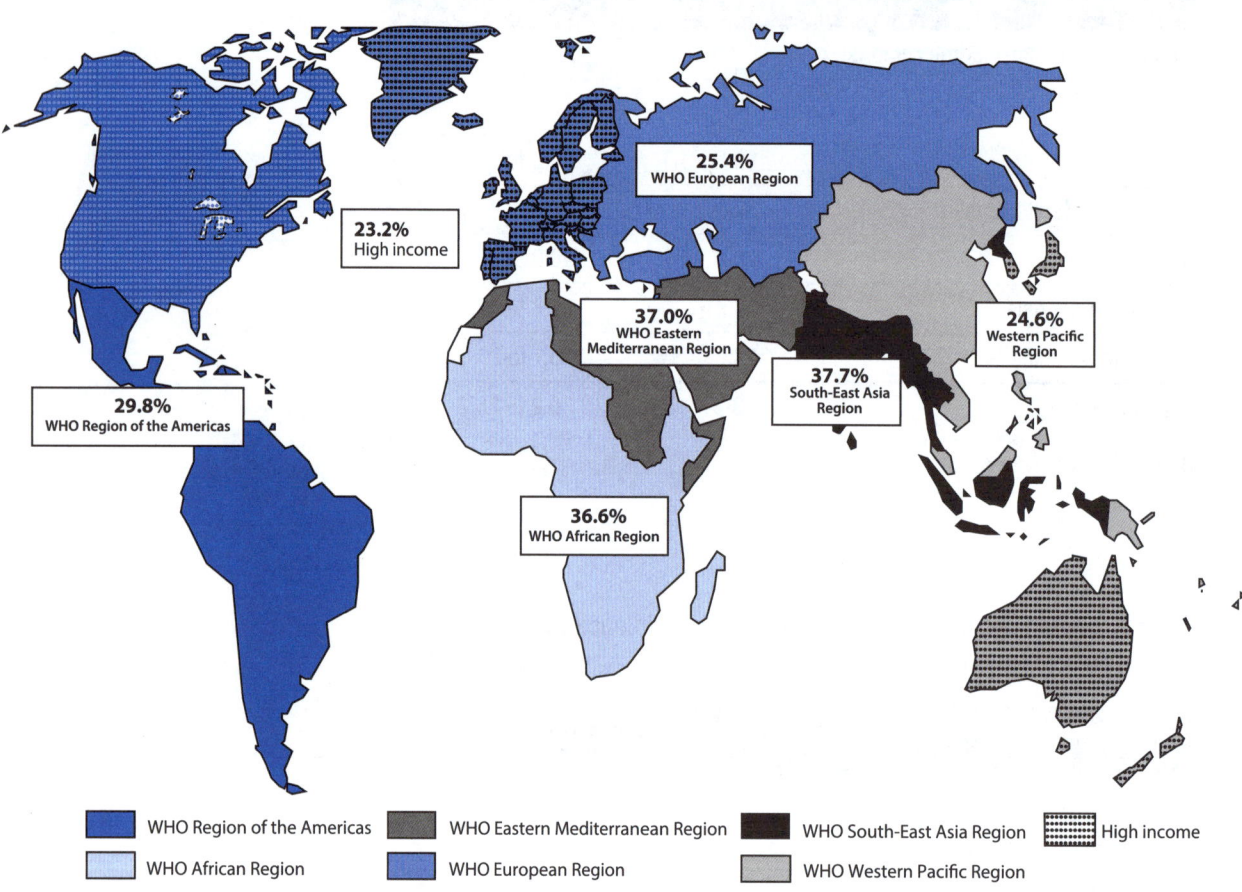

Figure 2. Global map showing regional prevalence rates of intimate partner violence by WHO region* (2010)

* Regional prevalence rates are presented for each WHO region including low- and middle-income countries, with high income countries analyzed separately. See Appendix 1 for list of countries with data available by region.

Global and regional prevalence estimates of non-partner sexual violence

The adjusted lifetime prevalence of non-partner sexual violence by region, based on data from 56 countries and two territories, is presented in Table 4. Globally, 7.2% (95% CI = 5.3% to 9.1%) of women reported ever having experienced non-partner sexual violence. There were variations across the WHO regions. The highest lifetime prevalence of non-partner sexual violence was reported in the high-income region (12.6%; 95% CI = 8.9% to 16.2%) and the African Region (11.9%; 95% CI = 8.5% to 15.3%), while the lowest prevalence was found for the South-East Asia Region (4.9%; 95% CI = 0.9% to 8.9%).

These differences between regions may arise for many reasons, and need to be interpreted with caution, especially as most of the regional estimates have wide confidence intervals. As well as real differences in the prevalence of non-partner sexual violence, the figures are likely to be subject to differing degrees of under-reporting by region. Sexual violence remains highly stigmatized in all settings, and even when studies take great care to address the sensitivity of the topic, it is likely that the levels of disclosure will be influenced by respondents' perceptions about the level of stigma associated with any disclosure, and the perceived repercussions of others knowing about this violence.

> The global lifetime prevalence of non-partner sexual violence is 7.2% (95% CI = 5.3% to 9.1%).

Age-specific prevalence rates are not included because of the lack of availability of age-specific data.

Table 4. Lifetime prevalence of non-partner sexual violence by WHO region

WHO region	Prevalence, %[a]	95% CI, %
Low- and middle-income regions:		
Africa	11.9	8.5 to 15.3
Americas	10.7	7.0 to 14.4
Eastern Mediterranean[b]	–	–
Europe	5.2	0.8 to 9.7
South-East Asia	4.9	0.9 to 8.9
Western Pacific	6.8	1.6 to 12.0
High income	12.6	8.9 to 16.2

CI = confidence interval.

[a] Results adjusted for interviewer training, whether the study was national and whether response options were broad enough to allow for different categories of perpetrators or were limited to a single category of perpetrator.

[b] No data were found for countries in this region, therefore a prevalence estimate is not provided

The prevalence of non-partner sexual violence among conflict-affected countries is an important aspect of the analysis, and data specific to conflict settings were identified (25, 26, 30–34, 43). However, these data were not analysed separately because data were only available from six conflict-affected countries and there was a high amount of variability in the sampling methodology, with several of the studies using population-based surveys of the entire country and others sampling specifically in conflict-affected regions. The lowest prevalence was reported from estimates from two large multi-country studies (IVAWS and GENACIS), while the higher prevalence estimates were from studies that focused on measuring violence in conflict-affected settings. It is often difficult to conduct population-based studies in conflict-affected settings, and obtaining a truly representative sample may be difficult because of logistical or security issues.

This review brings to light the lack of data on non-partner sexual violence in the general population as well as in conflict-affected settings. As compared to intimate partner violence, fewer studies include questions on non-partner sexual violence, there are more regions and countries for which no data are available, and it is not clear whether the questions being used generate accurate disclosure. While both forms of violence remain stigmatized, which impacts reporting, in many settings sexual violence is even more stigmatized, resulting in self-blame and shame, and disclosure may even put women's lives at risk. In addition, the measurement of intimate partner violence is more advanced than that of non-partner sexual violence, and there is more agreement among researchers on how to measure it.

Although we are aware that the data for non-partner sexual violence were not as robust or extensive as for intimate partner violence, it is likely that the differences in prevalence of non-partner sexual violence as compared to intimate partner violence reflect actual differences. It appears that intimate partner violence, which includes sexual violence, is considerably more prevalent and more common than non-partner sexual violence, as shown consistently in all regions.

When considering non-partner sexual violence in the context of violence against women and interpersonal violence in general, it appears that sexual violence is normative in settings where violence is common. As was seen in the *WHO multi-country study on women's health and domestic violence against women* (*21*), certain countries that had higher levels of non-partner sexual violence (Namibia and the United Republic of Tanzania), compared to others that had lower levels (Ethiopia), tended also to have higher rates of other forms of violence, such as sexual abuse during childhood (a form of non-partner sexual violence) and men fighting with other men.

Combined estimates of the prevalence of intimate partner violence and non-partner violence

Globally, 35.6% of women have ever experienced either non-partner sexual violence or physical or sexual violence by an intimate partner, or both.

While there are many other forms of violence that women are exposed to, the two forms studied here together represent a large proportion of the violence women experience globally. The global combined estimate demonstrates just how common physical and sexual violence is in the lives of many women.

Regional estimates show prevalence rates of intimate partner violence and non-partner sexual violence combined ranging from 27.2% to 45.6% (see Table 5).

Table 5. Lifetime prevalence of intimate partner violence (physical and/or sexual) or non-partner sexual violence or both among all women (15 years and older) by WHO region

WHO region	Proportion of women reporting intimate partner violence and/or non-partner sexual violence, %
Low- and middle-income regions:	
Africa	45.6
Americas	36.1
Eastern Mediterranean	36.4
Europe	27.2
South-East Asia	40.2
Western Pacific	27.9[a]
High income	32.7

[a] More recent studies from the Western Pacific Region using the WHO study methodology have since been published, but were not available at the time the data were compiled. They show very high prevalence rates of physical and/or sexual intimate partner violence between 60% and 68% (*40–42*).

Section 3: Results – the health effects of intimate partner violence and non-partner sexual violence

New systematic reviews were conducted on a broad range of health effects of exposure to intimate partner violence and non-partner sexual violence. For each of these reviews, extensive searches of electronic databases were carried out, including African Healthline, Applied Social Sciences Index and Abstracts, *British Medical Journal*, British Nursing Index, the Cochrane Library, CINAHL, Embase, Health Management Information Consortium, IMEMR, IMSEAR, International Bibliography of Social Sciences, LILACS, MedCarib, Midwives Information and Resource Service, NHS Library for Health Specialist Libraries, Ovid Medline, Popline, PsychINFO, PubMed, Science Direct, Web of Science, Wiley InterScience and WPRIM.

These reviews sought to include all published and unpublished studies that provided data on the strength of association between the different forms of violence considered and each health outcome. In general, no restriction on language or year of publication was specified. Cross-sectional, case-control and cohort studies in any population were eligible for review. All author definitions of violence were included, and the measures of exposures used were recorded, along with other indicators of the study's quality, and details of the factors controlled for in the analyses. In each case, relevant data were extracted using a standardized form. Random effects meta-analyses were used to generate pooled odds ratios for intimate partner violence where appropriate. For the health effects of non-partner sexual violence, pooled odds ratios were not generated, as there was too much variation in the definitions and measurements used. In these cases, best estimates from the literature are presented instead.

Health effects of exposure to intimate partner violence

This section describes the magnitude of the association between intimate partner violence and selected health outcomes: incident HIV infection, incident sexually transmitted infections (STIs), induced abortion, low birth weight, premature birth, growth restriction in utero and/or small for gestational age, alcohol use, depression and suicide, injuries, and death from homicide (Figure 1).

It is important to note that the selected outcomes presented here do not reflect the full range of health effects of exposure to intimate partner violence. For those that were chosen for this analysis, reasons included that there was at least some evidence from longitudinal studies, and sufficient published or raw data available to conduct a robust analysis in multiple settings, with at least some of the evidence coming from low- or middle-income countries; at least one of the studies included in the meta-analysis demonstrating a temporal order, with the violence clearly preceding the health risk; and plausible pathways of causality and mechanisms by which intimate partner violence can cause the selected outcome described in the literature. Results of the included health effects are summarized in Table 6 near the end of this section.

Other physical, mental and sexual and reproductive health effects have been linked with intimate partner violence, and merit similar attention, despite their exclusion from this report. These include adolescent pregnancy, unintended pregnancy in general, miscarriage, stillbirth, intrauterine haemorrhage, nutritional deficiency, abdominal pain and other gastrointestinal problems, neurological disorders, chronic pain, disability, anxiety and post-traumatic stress disorder (PTSD), as well as noncommunicable diseases such as hypertension, cancer and cardiovascular diseases. In addition, there is evidence linking intimate partner violence with negative child health and development outcomes, but these are not included in this report.

HIV and other sexually transmitted infections

Over the past decade, there has been growing recognition that intimate partner violence is an important contributor to women's vulnerability to HIV and STIs (*45–49*). The mechanisms underpinning a woman's increased vulnerability to HIV or STIs include direct infection from forced sexual intercourse, as well as the potential for increased risk from the general effects of prolonged exposure to stress (*49, 50*). Women in violent relationships, or who live in fear of violence, may also have limited control over the timing or circumstances of sexual intercourse, or their ability to negotiate condom use (*51*). Partner violence may also be an important determinant of separation, which in turn may increase a woman's risk of HIV if she acquires a new partner. Furthermore, there is behavioural evidence that men who use violence against their female partners are more likely than non-violent men to have a number of HIV-risk behaviours, including having multiple sexual partners (*52*), frequent alcohol use (*53*), visiting sex workers (*54*), and having an STI (*55, 56*), all of which can increase women's risk of HIV.

Forty-one studies were identified for inclusion in the review commissioned for this report (*57*). These included cohort, case-control and cross-sectional studies. The strongest evidence comes from cohort studies that use biological outcome measures, and allow determination of whether violence precedes incident HIV/STI infection. For this reason, although all of the evidence found was extracted, the analysis placed the most emphasis on the findings from cohort studies. Through the search, five cohort studies were found. Four of these explored the relationship between exposure to intimate partner violence and incident HIV or other STI infection. Two estimates looking at HIV infection and incident partner violence were also obtained. It was not possible to pool the findings because different measures were reported in different studies; we therefore propose best estimates based on the available studies. Of the studies of incident HIV/STI, the three large studies (*58–60*) (> 1000 participants) (two on HIV from sub-Saharan Africa and one on STI from India) found an increased risk of HIV/STI among those reporting partner violence. The fourth study (*61*), among women attending substance-use treatment clinics in the USA, used self-reported data on HIV and STI diagnosis, and found some evidence of a lower risk of HIV among those reporting intimate partner violence. The two studies looking at incident intimate partner violence (*61, 62*) (after HIV or STI diagnosis) found inconsistent results. The best estimates of association between intimate partner violence and HIV/STIs are odds ratio (OR) = 1.52 (95% CI = 1.03 to 2.23) for HIV (*58*); adjusted odds ratio (aOR) = 1.61 (95% CI = 1.24 to 2.08) for syphilis (*63*), and OR = 1.81 (95% CI = 0.90 to 3.63) for chlamydia or gonorrhea (*59*).

The review findings highlight the need for further research. Larger and more representative cohort studies from Africa and India show an association between experience of intimate partner violence and biologically confirmed incident HIV/other STIs. However, one smaller, lower-quality cohort study from a population with high competing risks for HIV infection showed an inverse relationship. Evidence from a broader range of settings is needed, to assess the degree to which the association between exposure to violence and incident HIV is also found in other HIV epidemic settings.

Induced abortion

Violent relationships are frequently marked by fear and controlling behaviours by partners, so it is not surprising that women in these relationships report more adverse sexual and reproductive health outcomes. The higher rates of adverse reproductive events can be explained by direct consequences of sexual violence and coercion, as well as by more indirect pathways affecting contraceptive use, such as sabotage of birth control, disapproval of birth control preventing use of contraception, or inability to negotiate condom use for fear of violence (*64*). As a result, women in abusive relationships have more unintended pregnancies (*65–67*). Of the estimated 80 million unintended pregnancies each year, at least half are terminated through induced abortion (*68*) and nearly half of those take place in unsafe conditions (*69*). While unintended pregnancies carried to term have been associated with health risk to mothers and infants, illegal and unsafe abortions place women's health at even greater risk.

Analysis of data from 31 studies provides strong evidence that women with a history of intimate partner violence are more likely to report having had an induced abortion (pooled OR = 2.16, 95% CI = 1.88 to 2.49). Similar results were found in a subanalysis of five studies in which it could be confirmed that intimate partner violence preceded the abortion (OR = 2.38, 95% CI = 1.93 to 2.84). The effect of other factors, such as the timing of violence and legality of abortion were also explored, and explain some of the heterogeneity in estimates (*70*).

The review confirmed that higher rates of induced abortion among women with a history of intimate partner violence are consistently found in a variety of study designs and among diverse population groups. Sensitive and stigmatized events, such as abortion, tend to be underreported, particularly in settings where it is illegal, but the inclusion of case-control studies involving abortion patients provided important evidence of association. These findings emphasize the importance of addressing intimate partner violence in health settings, particularly in sexual and reproductive health services.

Low birth weight and prematurity

Low birth weight can result from either preterm birth or growth restriction *in utero*, both of which can be directly linked to stress. Living in an abusive and dangerous environment marked by chronic stress can therefore be an important risk factor for maternal health, as well as affecting birth weight.

All observational studies (cohort, case-control, and cross-sectional) that investigated intimate partner violence and the potential association with low birth weight/preterm birth/growth restriction *in utero* were considered. Only studies for which the perpetrator was limited to the intimate partner and for which violence was limited to physical and/or sexual were eligible for review. Low birth weight was defined as < 2500 g, preterm birth was defined as gestational age of less than 37 weeks, and growth restriction *in utero* and/or small for gestational age was defined as birth weight below the tenth percentile.

A total of 17 studies met the inclusion criteria (13 low birth weight, 10 preterm birth, 3 growth restriction *in utero*). Intimate partner violence was positively associated with low birth weight (aOR = 1.16, 95% CI = 1.02 to 1.29), as was preterm birth (aOR = 1.41, 95% CI = 1.21 to 1.62), even after adjusting for confounding factors. No statistically significant association was found between intimate partner violence and intrauterine growth restriction (aOR = 1.36, 95% CI = 0.53 to 2.19). Heterogeneity scores were statistically significant in the analysis of low birth weight, but they were much lower for growth restriction *in utero* and preterm birth *(71)*.

Given the known causal mechanisms of stress-related responses affecting birth weight and the consistent positive association found, these results suggest that intimate partner violence is indeed an important risk factor for having low-birth-weight babies.

Harmful alcohol use

Harmful use of alcohol and violence are intertwined. As well as alcohol being an important facilitator of men's use of violence, there is also evidence of an association for women between violence and frequent alcohol use. The nature of this association is likely to be complex. Women may drink alcohol to cope with the sequelae of abuse, but, conversely, women's consumption of alcohol may result in abuse from their partners, for example, because their partners believe that they should not drink.

The review identified a total of 37 studies, providing 77 estimates of association between physical and/or sexual intimate partner violence and alcohol use.

Six longitudinal studies, with 10 estimates, examined whether intimate partner violence was associated with incident alcohol use. All of these longitudinal estimates showed a positive direction of association between intimate partner violence and incident alcohol use, although not all were statistically significant *(72)*. The best estimate from the available literature is from a longitudinal study on women's health in Australia, in which alcohol abuse was measured subsequent to disclosure of intimate partner violence. This study reported an OR of 1.82 (95% CI = 1.04 to 3.18) *(73)*.

Overall, longitudinal studies illustrate that the relationship between alcohol use and violence is bidirectional. There is a positive association between women's experience of intimate partner violence and subsequent alcohol use, as well as an association between alcohol use and subsequent intimate partner violence. Although the causal relationship between experience of intimate partner violence and alcohol consumption in women is far from clear, there is clear evidence that women with histories of violence consume more alcohol, and, conversely, that women who binge drink and consume alcohol in other harmful ways are more likely to report experiences of violence. It is also possible that both alcohol use and intimate partner violence can be attributed to another underlying issue, such as a mental health disorder or another substance use, which can increase women's vulnerability to violence and to alcohol use. Public health programming needs to address alcohol use in prevention and treatment of intimate partner violence, and experiences of violence need to be addressed in alcohol misuse programmes.

Depression and suicide

Traumatic stress is thought to be the main mechanism that explains why intimate partner violence may cause subsequent depression and suicide attempts. Exposures to traumatic events can lead to stress, fear and isolation, which, in turn, may lead to depression and suicidal behaviour *(74)*. Again, the relationship may be bidirectional: other studies suggest that women with severe mental health difficulties are more likely to experience violent victimization *(75, 76)*. Developmental and early life exposures to violence and other traumas may also play an important role in predicting both violence and depression *(77, 78)*.

Seventeen papers were identified, reporting on 16 studies, giving a total of 36 163 participants, and containing 55 effect estimates *(79)*. For violence and incident depression, the pooled OR from six studies was 1.97 (95% CI = 1.56 to 2.48). There was some heterogeneity[5] between studies (I^2 = 50.4%, P = 0.073), but all estimates but one showed a positive direction of effect. Three studies (*80–82*) examined violence and subsequent suicide attempts. All three showed positive relationships; two were statistically significant and one was borderline significant. A pooled OR of 4.54 (95% CI = 1.78 to 11.61) was calculated from these three studies (*80–82*).

Non-fatal injuries

Intimate partner violence is associated with many health consequences, but the most direct effects are fatal and non-fatal physical injuries. It is estimated that approximately half of women in abusive relationships in the USA are physically injured by their partners, and that most of them sustain multiple types of injuries (*83*). The head, neck and face are the most common locations of injuries related to partner violence, followed by musculoskeletal injuries and genital injuries. Measurement of injuries resulting from intimate partner violence remains challenging for many reasons.

Unlike other health effects of violence, measuring the relative risk of injury among women experiencing intimate partner violence as compared to women with no partner violence is less relevant and generally not feasible. Practically speaking, studies do not quantify injuries among women who are not experiencing partner violence, and therefore relative risks were not presented or were not calculable in most of the studies. A more practical measure of interest in understanding the health effects of intimate partner violence is the prevalence of injury directly attributable to partner violence, not the relative rate of injury among women experiencing and not experiencing partner violence. The few studies for which this relative risk information was available were analysed, and the relative risk data are presented below. Population-based surveys, such as the DHS in countries that included a module on intimate partner violence with questions inquiring about physical injuries due to violence, complement these sources of data and provide a more direct estimate of injuries due to violence. These population-based data can be considered a more reliable and valid data source for these purposes, since they capture treated as well as untreated injuries that can be directly attributable to partner violence (because of the wording used in the surveys, which asks women who have experienced intimate partner violence whether they sustained injuries from the violence). The self-reported nature of the results, and the potential recall bias when time has elapsed, can bias the findings; however, given the limitations of the different data sources, the population-based studies provide more direct estimates of better quality.

Hospital- and clinic-based data were not included in this analysis, since surveillance data from clinics or hospitals, when available, vastly underestimate injuries due to violence for several reasons: many women, regardless of health systems in their country, do not seek health care for injuries

---

5. In meta-analyses, tests of heterogeneity (e.g. I^2) are used to show how much the individual studies show variability as opposed to consistency of results across studies. Higher heterogeneity scores that are statistically significant indicate that the variability is not due to chance alone.

caused by partner violence (*84*),[6] and if they do, many or most hospitals do not collect perpetrator information. Furthermore, even when asked about perpetrators, women presenting with injuries due to partner violence may be reluctant to disclose the actual source of the injury, attributing the injury to some other cause.

Random effects meta-analysis was conducted to summarize the data extracted from the 11 papers and data from the 31 countries with population-based data (*85*). The proportion of women with injuries due to intimate partner violence among all women who had experienced partner violence was 41.8% (95% CI = 34.0% to 49.6%; weighting based on inverse variance). The relative risk of injuries for women with and without intimate partner violence was calculated where data allowed (i.e. three studies (*86–88*) for which injury rates among women without and women with partner violence were presented), showing an OR of 2.92 (95% CI = 2.21 to 3.63). Despite the serious limitations in the published data, the results from the population-based studies added strength to the analysis, by analysing data from women in the general population. These results, indicating that among women experiencing intimate partner violence 42% were injured by their partners, shows the potentially enormous health burden for women as a result of injuries from intimate partner violence.

Fatal injuries (intimate partner homicides)

Two methods were used to obtain estimates of the proportion of male and female homicides where the perpetrator was an intimate partner. First, a systematic review of all published and unpublished studies released between 1 January 1994 and 31 December 2011 found 2167 abstracts, of which 118 studies that examined the proportion of intimate partner homicides were included. Second, a survey was conducted among 169 countries with official data sources and relevant web pages or contact information to gather country- or regional-level data on intimate partner homicide. Contact was made via e-mail with the country statistics offices, ministries of justice, home offices, or police headquarters, if relevant information could not be found on home pages. In total, 226 different studies and statistics were found, capturing 1121 estimates across 65 countries from 1982 to 2011 (*89*).

For the total estimates, the total numbers of homicides by intimate partners were added by sex and divided by the total homicides by sex. Since some estimates are skewed, the findings are reported in median percentages. Regional estimates are given according to WHO regions.

Across all countries with available data since 1982:

- the median prevalence of intimate partner homicide was approximately 13%, with as many as 38% of all murdered women (in contrast to 6% of all murdered men) being killed by an intimate partner;

- the median prevalence of intimate partner homicide among all murdered women was highest in the South-East Asia Region, with approximately 55%, and the high-income region, with approximately 41%, followed by the African Region (approximately 40%) and the Region of the Americas (approximately 38%).

The regional differences in intimate partner homicide may represent real differences in patterns of homicide and correspond with the cultural acceptability of violence against women and the

---

6. Data from the *WHO multi-country study on women's health and domestic violence against women (21)* confirmed this finding, with data from 14 sites in 9 countries. While, on average, 48% of women experiencing physical intimate partner violence claimed they needed health care for their injuries, only 36% actually sought health care for them.

prevalence of intimate partner violence against women. However, the regional differences may also be closely correlated with the completeness and quality of data on homicides among countries and regions, as there is a lack of data on intimate partner homicide in low-income settings, especially in Asia and Africa, and a high amount of missing data on the victim–offender relationship in Latin America.

The prevalence rates of intimate partner homicide presented are likely to be underestimations, since the victim–offender relationship is often not known or reported. Over- or underestimations might have also occurred because the study was restricted to one estimate per country year, which was averaged if data for more than one year were available. In addition, the study favored national representative information over small-scale studies, which might have gone into more depth, for example through data triangulation, to establish the victim–offender relationship.

Table 6 summarizes the information on the effect sizes for selected health outcomes and intimate partner violence.

Health effects of exposure to non-partner sexual violence

The health effects of non-partner sexual violence – in particular the mental health effects (depression, anxiety disorders, including PTSD) are often referred to in reports and discussions. This review showed that population-based evidence on the strength of these associations is extremely limited. Currently, most evidence comes from clinical research and observation, rather than from longitudinal or case-control studies. Where the associations are measured, reports of sexual violence by all types of perpetrators (intimate and non-intimate partners) are often combined and were therefore not included. The reviews of the health effects associated with non-partner sexual violence reveal the poor state of research and highlight the need for dedicated longitudinal studies. No single longitudinal study or systematic review was found for any of the health associations with non-partner sexual violence. It was also found that health outcomes were not well defined and both the limited number of studies and the huge variations in the definitions used meant it was not possible to carry out a meta-analysis. The reviews conducted for mental health outcomes and harmful use of alcohol associated with non-partner sexual violence are summarized in the text below and in a summary table (Table 7) at the end of this section.

Depression and anxiety

Five studies, all based in the USA, were found to report associations between non-partner sexual violence and depression/anxiety disorders.

All studies found a positive association, but these were not consistently significant, nor did they consistently adjust for relevant factors. A large female veteran study of 137 006 women by Kimerling et al. (*90*), using the diagnostic categories of the *Diagnostic and statistical manual of mental disorders*, 4th edition (DSM-IV) (*91*), reported an adjusted OR of 2.25 (95% CI = 2.10 to 2.40), while a second, military-based study by Hankin et al. (*92*), using a shortened version of the Centre for Epidemiological Studies Depression scale (CES-D) (*93*) (11 items), reported an adjusted OR of 3.16 (95% CI = 2.68 to 3.72). The study by Kimerling et al. (*90*) adjusted for race, age, and knowing own medical/mental health condition, while the study by Hankin et al. (*92*) adjusted for age and educational level. It appears that neither of the two military studies adjusted for military trauma.

The 1998 Women's Survey (*94*) found a non-significant association between non-partner sexual violence and a high score of depression symptoms (OR = 1.25; 95% CI = 0.61 to 2.59), which was measured using a subscale from the CES-D scale. The cut-off for the high score was not provided. However, the same study also measured the association with a physician diagnosis of depression and/or anxiety within the last 5 years, and a significant association was reported (OR = 2.59; 95% CI = 1.17 to 5.72). This study adjusted for age, race, marital status, education and income. A similar positive association between depression and anxiety was found in a study of 1336 female university employees (*95*). This study used a modified CES-D scale to measure depression, and anxiety was measured using nine items from the Profile of Mood States scale (*96*), with adjustments for race, age and occupation. Finally, a study among 174 female patients (*97*) attending an internal medicine clinic and using the Hopkins checklist (*98*), reported an association between non-partner sexual violence and depression, with an adjusted OR of 2.5 (95% CI = 1.63 to 7.48).

Alcohol use disorders

A limited body of research and differing definitions made it impossible to conduct a meta-analysis of the available results. The literature search resulted in five eligible studies. These were all cross-sectional studies (six papers) reporting associations between non-partner sexual violence and alcohol use disorders, and will be described briefly here. Three of the studies are from the USA (*90, 92, 95, 99*: references (*95*) and (*99*) are reports on the same study), one from Switzerland (*100*) and one from Lima, Peru (*101*). Two of the studies are based on military samples (*90, 92*), two on samples from workers (*95, 99, 101*), and the Swiss study was among adolescent girls, aged 15 to 20 years, enrolled in schools or professional training programmes (*100*). All the studies except one (*101*) reported adjustments for variables such as age, race, occupation, employment income and marital status, while the study among workers also adjusted for work-related stress (*99*). The two military-sample studies did not report whether additional adjustments were made for work context, i.e. adjustments for military-related trauma.

There were many differences in what was considered as alcohol use problems in these studies, with the study by Kimerling et al. (*90*) reporting on alcohol use disorder, which was quantified according to the mental health and substance abuse clinical classification using the DSM-IV (*88*). Hankin et al. (*92*) measured "alcohol abuse", which was quantified using the five-item TWEAK scale (an acronym for the five questions used [T – Tolerance, W – Worried, E – Eye opener, A – Amnesia – black-outs, K – K/Cut down]. Rospenda et al. (*99*), reporting on the sample of university workers, measured associations between non-partner sexual violence and "problem drinking", using a combination of the Michigan Assessment Screening Test for Alcohol and Drugs scale (*102*) with one or more instances of drinking to intoxication and one or more instances of heavy episodic drinking. Heavy episodic drinking and drinking to intoxication was also measured in the study among adolescent girls (*95*), and was based on two questions. This study measured "drinking alcohol regularly", but detail on how this was measured was not provided. Similarly, the study among workers in Lima (*101*) presented measures of association between non-partner sexual violence with alcohol consumption but no detail was provided on how alcohol consumption was measured.

All six papers reported positive associations with non-partner sexual violence, with five reporting

Table 6. Summary of effect size estimates for selected health outcomes and intimate partner violence

Domain	Disease/injury resulting from violence	Definition	Search date	Number of studies identified	Effect size (95% CI)[a]
Sexual health	HIV/AIDS	Infection with HIV, with or without progression to AIDS	December 2010	17	OR = 1.52[b] (1.03 to 2.23)
	Syphilis infection	Acute and chronic infection with Treponema pallidum	December 2010	21	aOR = 1.61[c] (1.24 to 2.08)
	Chlamydia or gonorrhoea	Bacterial infection with Chlamydia trachomatis, transmitted vaginally, anally or perinatally;[d] Bacterial infection with Neisseria gonorrhoea, transmitted vaginally, anally or perinatally	December 2010	21	OR = 1.81[e] (0.90 to 3.63)
Reproductive health	Induced abortion	Episodes of induced abortion	December 2011	31	OR = 2.16[f] (1.88 to 2.49)
Perinatal health	Low birth weight	< 2500 g	June 2012	13	aOR = 1.16[g] (1.02 to 1.29)
	Premature birth	Gestational age < 37 weeks	June 2012	10	aOR = 1.41[g] (1.97 to 2.60)
	Small for gestational age	Birth weight below the 10th percentile	June 2012	3	aOR = 1.36[g] (0.53 to 2.19)
Mental health	Unipolar depressive disorders	Depressive episodes	February 2013	16	OR = 1.97[h] (1.56 to 2.48)
	Alcohol use disorders	Alcohol use disorders; authors' definitions	January 2011	36	OR = 1.82[i] (1.04 to 3.18)
Injuries	Any injury inflicted by partner	Injuries inflicted by partner	September 2011	11 papers + data from 31 countries	42% of women with intimate partner violence were injured by their partner (34% to 49.6%)[j] 2.92[k] (2.21 to 3.63), comparing injuries among women with and without intimate partner violence
Death	Homicide	Death perpetrated by partner	December 2011	226	Approximately 13% of all murders, 38% of all female murders and 6% of all male murders[l]
	Suicide	Death perpetrated by self	November 2011	3	OR = 4.54[m] (1.78 to 11.61)

[a] Effect size refers to the estimate of association and is based on either a best estimate from the literature or a pooled estimate from a meta-analysis.
[b] Best estimate (58).
[c] Best estimate (63).
[d] Excludes ocular trachoma.
[e] Best estimate (59).
[f] Pooled estimate (70).
[g] Pooled estimate (71).
[h] Pooled estimate from 6 studies (79).
[i] Best estimate (73).
[j] Pooled estimate (85).
[k] Pooled estimate from 3 studies (86–88).
[l] Pooled estimate (89).
[m] Pooled estimate (79)

significant associations: alcohol disorders OR = 2.33 (95% CI = 2.15 to 2.53) (*90*); alcohol consumption OR = 1.92 (95% CI = 1.62 to 2.38) (*101*); drinking to intoxication OR = 1.72 (95% CI = 1.26 to 2.36) (*95*); alcohol abuse OR = 1.89 (95% CI = 1.27 to 2.60) (*92*); and drinking alcohol regularly OR = 1.95 (95% CI = 1.5 to 2.5) (*100*). Despite the limitation of the estimates, it is clear that non-partner sexual violence is associated with problem alcohol use. In the absence of a pooled estimate, the estimate of "alcohol disorders" was used, which was based on the largest sample (n = 134 894) and which was also based on the DSM-IV (*91*) clinical classification of mental health disorders and conditions.

Table 7 summarizes the effect size for depression and alcohol use disorders and non-partner sexual violence against women.

Table 7. **Summary of effect size estimates for depression and alcohol use disorders and non-partner sexual violence**

Domain	Disease/injury resulting from violence	Definition	Search date	Number of studies identified	Effect size (95% CI)[a]
Mental health	Unipolar depressive disorders combined with:	Depressive episodes	May 2012	5	OR = 2.59[b] (1.17 to 5.72)
	Anxiety disorders	Including PTSD and obsessive–compulsive disorder	May 2012		
	Alcohol use disorders		May 2012	5	OR = 2.33[c] (2.15 to 2.53)

a Effect size refers to the estimate of association and is based on either a best estimate from the literature.

b Best estimate (94).

c Best estimate (90).

Section 4: Summary and conclusions

Summary of findings

This comprehensive review of the prevalence and health effects of two forms of violence against women (intimate partner violence and non-partner sexual violence) marks an important milestone, not only in the field of research in violence against women, but also in the field of public health in general. This report presents the first global and regional prevalence estimates of physical and sexual intimate partner violence against women, and non-partner sexual violence against women, using evidence from comprehensive systematic reviews of global population data.

The findings confirm the fact that intimate partner violence and non-partner sexual violence are widespread and affect women throughout the world. Despite this evidence, many still choose to view the violent experiences of women as disconnected events, taking place in the private sphere of relationship conflict and beyond the realm of policy-makers and health-care providers. Others blame the women themselves for being subjected to violence, rather than the perpetrators. In the case of non-partner sexual violence, women are blamed for deviating from accepted social roles, for being in the wrong place, or for wearing the wrong clothes. In the case of partner violence, women are blamed for talking to another man, refusing sexual intercourse, not asking permission from their partner (e.g., for going out, visiting their family), or for not conforming to their role as wives/ partners in some other way.

The health sector in particular has been slow to engage with violence against women. Yet, this report presents clear evidence that exposure to violence is an important determinant of poor health for women. This is in spite of the fact that this report has only looked at a limited set of health outcomes.

The findings highlight that intimate partner violence is a major contributor to women's mental health problems, particularly depression and suicidality, as well as to sexual and reproductive health problems, including maternal health and neonatal health problems.

Globally 35.6% have experienced either intimate partner violence and/or non-partner sexual violence. Nearly one third of ever-partnered women (30.0%) have experienced physical and/or sexual violence by an intimate partner, and 7.2% of adult women have experienced sexual violence by a non-partner. Some women have experienced both.

Key findings on health outcomes of physical and sexual intimate partner violence include:

- globally, as many as 38% of all murders of women are reported as being committed by intimate partners;

- 42% of women who have been physically and/or sexually abused by a partner have experienced injuries as a result of that violence;

- women who have experienced partner violence have higher rates of several important health problems and risk behaviours; compared to women who have not experienced partner violence, they:

  – have 16% greater odds of having a low-birth-weight baby;

  – are more than twice as likely to have an induced abortion;

  – are more than twice as likely to experience depression;

- in some regions, they are 1.5 times more likely to acquire HIV, and 1.6 times more likely to have syphilis,[7] compared to women who do not suffer partner violence.

---

7. This association was found for sexual intimate partner violence only.

The review confirms the degree to which women with violent partners may be injured. However, despite injury often being perceived to be one of the outcomes of intimate partner violence, the reviews found surprisingly limited data on this issue, with gaps in population data, particularly on the extent and forms of injury that women experience in different settings.

While, across regions, there are consistently higher rates of intimate partner violence than non-partner sexual violence, this does not indicate that non-partner sexual violence should be given less attention or be seen as less significant to women's health. We know that sexual violence remains highly stigmatized, and carries heavy social sanctions in many settings. Furthermore, given the sensitivities of reporting sexual violence, we know these estimates are likely to underestimate actual prevalence. While measures of partner violence capture a spectrum of acts of physical, sexual and psychological[8] violence, ranging from less severe to the most severe forms of violence, sexual violence, by definition, is among the most severe forms of violence.

The fact that, in spite of the constraints to reporting, 7.2% of women globally have reported non-partner sexual violence provides important evidence of the extent of this problem. This review found that women who have experienced non-partner sexual violence are 2.3 times more likely to have alcohol use disorders and 2.6 times more likely to have depression or anxiety than women who have not experienced non-partner sexual violence.

This is supported by clinical experience, which shows that sexual violence can profoundly affect physical and mental health in the short and long term, contributing to the burden of ill health among survivors. Some studies have shown that women who have been raped have higher rates of use of medical care (e.g. visits to the doctor, hospitalizations) compared to women who have not been raped, even years after the event (*103*). These data also highlight the need to find better ways to help the survivors of sexual violence and prevent more women and girls from suffering these experiences in the first place.

Limitations of the review

The review was constrained by the availability of data, and, in particular, of data of sufficient quality to assess the health burden of both intimate partner violence and sexual violence by perpetrators other than partners. It also only looked at a selected number of health outcomes, and was unable to assess the level of comorbidity; women suffering intimate partner violence, in particular, are likely to be experiencing more than one health outcome at a point in time.

The estimates of prevalence and health burden were limited to physical and sexual intimate partner violence and did not include emotional/psychological abuse, even though qualitative research shows this to be an important element of intimate partner violence, which many women report as being particularly disabling and resulting in ill health. There is a need to strengthen methodologies for measuring this type of violence, testing them cross-culturally and developing consensus on them.

The review has highlighted the data gap in relation to non-partner sexual violence, and, in particular, the need for improving the way in which results from studies of sexual violence are reported. This is most evident in the absence of population

---

8. This review did not include psychological/emotional violence, as there are fewer data available and much more variation in how this is measured across studies.

data from conflict settings, in spite of the growing attention to this issue.

This report also only considers measures of sexual violence among women aged 15 years or more. If sexual violence in all of its forms – by all perpetrators (partners and non-partners), during childhood and adulthood – were measured together, the prevalence rates would be much higher than those found here. Evidence also shows that women who have experienced one form of violence are more likely to experience another episode of violence, which would not be captured in an aggregated measure of sexual violence. While the global and regional prevalence estimates presented in this report are an important step in documenting the epidemiology of this public health problem, more information is needed to understand and document sexual violence more accurately.

This report has sought to quantify the health burden, but the bidirectional relationship with many factors makes this difficult, in the absence of high-quality longitudinal data where both the exposures to violence and the health outcomes are measured at multiple time points.

The number of health outcomes that were included in this review was limited for methodological, time and resource reasons. An important omission from the review was evidence on the relationship between exposures to intimate partner violence and noncommunicable diseases. There is research indicating a relationship with chronic conditions, including cardiovascular disease and hypertension (104) and we are beginning to understand better the potential pathways that explain these relationships (105). However, this was not addressed in this review. The review did look at the relationship with harmful use of alcohol, which, together with smoking (also not addressed in this review), is associated with cardiovascular and other noncommunicable diseases. The review also did not discuss the compelling literature on the effects of partner violence on child health and developmental and behavioural outcomes (106–109).

Implications of the findings

Research gaps

This work and these findings highlight several research gaps that must be noted in the interpretation of these data and that should inform future research.

First, the prevalence estimates highlight several gaps in population-based data. Many countries have not collected population-based data on either intimate partner violence or non-partner violence, and the prevalence rates for these countries are unknown. This was most evident in the total lack of data from the Eastern Mediterranean Region on non-partner sexual violence, making it impossible to calculate an estimate for this region. Looking at the regions in more detail (See Table A.2.1), the regions with the least data available on intimate partner violence were Central Sub-Saharan Africa, East Asia, Caribbean and Central Asia. Countries that do have data often base their estimates on inadequate survey instruments or methodologies. The gold standard for valid data on violence against women is currently a stand-alone specialized survey, such as the *WHO multi-country study on women's health and domestic violence against women* (21), with adequate measures taken to address the ethical and safety issues that are unique to this type of research. These measures include specialized training of female interviewers to collect data in a private space, in a non-judgmental manner, in the absence of male partners; provision of referrals if necessary; and interviewing only one woman per household, to prevent knowledge about the survey content being shared. The training of interviewers is also critical and when this is done appropriately, women are more likely to disclose their experiences of all forms of violence and are more likely to feel supported in their disclosure, particularly when adequate safety measures are taken. Other surveys, such as DHS also provide some of these safety measures when using the violence against women module but, in general, violence modules added to other surveys tend to achieve lower disclosure rates, thereby reducing the overall prevalence rates documented.

Second, less is known about how to capture experiences of sexual violence. Questions on intimate partner violence have received more attention and the measurement of partner violence is more advanced in terms of which questions to ask and how to capture exposure to partner violence, particularly physical and, less so, sexual partner violence. Revisions have been made or are under way in several large violence survey instruments (4, 21), which will improve measurement, and can serve as a model for other surveys on violence. It is less clear whether the current questions used to capture experiences of non-partner sexual violence adequately capture the range of these experiences. Not only do the actual questions on sexual violence need improvement and further validation, but multiple experiences and multiple perpetrators over different time periods are important aspects of sexual violence that also need to be captured adequately. These measurement issues are particularly relevant for conflict settings, where this review has shown a large gap in robust data.

Third, it is important to note that differences in political and cultural factors mean that individual countries need their own data, and that extrapolating one country's prevalence estimates to another is not necessarily appropriate for policy and programmatic decision-making. So, while two countries might share a border and might have cultural and other similarities, and the experience of violence against women may be assumed to be the same in the two places, each country will need to collect its own data, in order to understand the risk factors related to violence against women in that particular context and to respond appropriately. Collecting sound data on the magnitude and nature of the problem has served in many countries as a stimulus to acknowledge and name the problem and initiate discussions on policies and strategies to address it. This will also provide a baseline against which countries can measure progress.

Finally, the data on health effects are predominantly based on cross-sectional studies, although the analyses in this report preferentially used effect estimates from longitudinal research, where these were available. Proving causality without establishing temporality is not possible, although other evidence is provided to support a causal hypothesis for these outcomes. For example:

- the causal pathways outlined in the conceptual framework in Figure 1 provide theoretical grounding in biological and behavioural mechanisms through which intimate partner violence can lead to selected health outcomes;

- the review replicates findings in a variety of settings, using population-based surveys;

- the review establishes temporal relationships for some of the findings, such as some of the studies in the intimate partner violence and abortion analysis and the intimate partner violence and low birth weight/prematurity analyses, since pregnancy outcomes were recorded by researchers at the time of the study and reports of partner violence would have preceded these outcomes;

- in some of the analyses, the review establishes a dose–response association, with more severe outcomes found among more severely abused women;

- most importantly, the review finds strong, statistically significant associations when data are pooled for each of these outcomes, even after adjusting for confounding factors.

The review has maximized the use of the available data, but stronger conclusions could be made if more longitudinal data were available, if biological markers were available for some health issues, and if more studies controlled for relevant confounding factors. Better study designs would enable greater understanding of the nature of the health effects of intimate partner violence and non-partner sexual violence.

Conclusions

In light of these data, in which more than one in three women (35.6%) globally report having experienced physical and/or sexual partner violence, or sexual violence by a non-partner, the evidence is incontrovertible – violence against women is a public health problem of epidemic proportions. It pervades all corners of the globe, puts women's health at risk, limits their participation in society, and causes great human suffering.

The findings underpin the need for the health sector to take intimate partner violence and sexual violence against women more seriously. All health-care providers should be trained to understand the relationship between violence and women's ill health and to be able to respond appropriately. Multiple entry points within the health sector exist where women may seek health care – without necessarily disclosing violence – particularly in sexual and reproductive health services (e.g. antenatal care, post-abortion care, family planning), mental health and emergency services. The new WHO guidelines for the health sector response to intimate partner violence and sexual violence (110) emphasize the urgent need to integrate these issues into undergraduate curricula for all health-care providers, as well as in in-service training.

In relation to sexual violence, whether by a partner or non-partner, access to comprehensive post-rape care is essential, and must ideally happen within 72 hours. The new WHO guidelines (110) describe this as including first-line psychological support, emergency contraception, prophylaxis for HIV, diagnosis and prophylaxis for other STIs, and short- and long-term mental health support. This should also include access to collection and analysis of forensic evidence for those women who choose to follow a judicial procedure. Similarly, for intimate partner violence, access to first-line psychological support, mental health and other support services needs to be developed and strengthened.

This health sector response needs to be part of a multisectoral response, as recently endorsed in the Agreed Conclusions of the 57th session of the Commission on the Status of Women (2). The Commission makes recommendations for and urges governments and other actors, at all levels, to:

- strengthen the implementation of legal and policy frameworks and accountability;

- address structural and underlying causes and risk factors, in order to prevent violence against women and girls;

- strengthen multisectoral services, programmes and responses to violence against women and girls.

The high prevalence of these forms of violence against women globally, and in all regions, also highlights the need to go beyond services and the importance of working simultaneously on preventing this violence from happening in the first place. The variation in the prevalence of violence seen within and between communities, countries and regions highlights that violence is not inevitable, and that it can be prevented.

There is growing evidence about the factors that explain much of the global variation. This evidence highlights the need to address the economic and sociocultural factors that foster a culture of violence against women. Promising prevention programmes exist, particularly for intimate partner violence, and need to be tested and scaled up. Interventions for prevention include: challenging social norms that support male authority and control over women and that condone violence against women; reducing levels of childhood exposure to violence; reforming discriminatory family law; strengthening women's economic rights; eliminating gender inequalities in access to formal wage employment and secondary education (*111, 112*); and, at an individual level, addressing harmful use of alcohol. Growing evidence from surveys of men asking about perpetration of rape/sexual assault against non-partners, and physical and sexual violence against partners, also points to the need to address social and cultural norms around masculinity, gender power relationships and violence. (*113, 114*)

This report unequivocally demonstrates that violence against women is pervasive globally and that it is a major contributing factor to women's ill health. In combination, these findings send a powerful message that violence against women is not a small problem that only occurs in some pockets of society, but rather is a global public health problem of epidemic proportions, requiring urgent action. As recently endorsed by the Commission on the Status of Women (*2*), it is time for the world to take action: a life free of violence is a basic human right, one that every woman, man and child deserves.

References

1. *Report of the Fourth World Conference on Women*. New York, United Nations, 1995 (A/CONF.177/20/Rev.1) (http://www.un.org/womenwatch/confer/beijing/reports/, accessed 1 April 2013).

2. The elimination and prevention of all forms of violence against women and girls: agreed conclusions. In: *Commission on the Status of Women*, Fifty-seventh session, 4–15 March 2013. New York, United Nations, 2013 (http://www.un.org/womenwatch/daw/csw/57sess.htm, accessed 1 April 2013).

3. Department of Gender and Women's Health Family and Community Health, World Health Organization. *Putting women's safety first: ethical and safety recommendations for research on domestic violence against women.* Geneva, World Health Organization, 2001 (WHO/FCH/GWH/01.1).

4. Measure DHS Demographic and Health Surveys. *DHS questionnaire modules* (English, French) (http://www.measuredhs.com/publications/publication-dhsqm-dhs-questionnaires-and-manuals.cfm, accessed 1 April 2013).

5. Centers for Disease Control and Prevention. Reproductive health surveys (http://www.cdc.gov/reproductivehealth/Global/surveys.htm, accessed 1 April 2013).

6. Krug EG et al., eds. *World report on violence and health*. Geneva, World Health Organization, 2002.

7. Black MC, Breiding MJ. Adverse health conditions and health risk behaviors associated with intimate partner violence – United States, 2005. *Morbidity and Mortality Weekly Report,* 2008, 57(5):113–117.

8. Black MC. Intimate partner violence and adverse health consequences. *American Journal of Lifestyle Medicine*, 2011, 5(5):428–439.

9. Howard LM et al. Domestic violence and severe psychiatric disorders: prevalence and interventions. *Psychological Medicine*, 2010, 40(6):881–893.

10. Miller AH. Neuroendocrine and immune system interactions in stress and depression. *Psychiatric Clinics of North America*, 1998, 21(2):443–463.

11. Altarac M, Strobino D. Abuse during pregnancy and stress because of abuse during pregnancy and birthweight. *Journal of the American Medical Women's Association*, 2002, 57(4):208–214.

12. Wadhwa PD, Entinger S, Buss C, Lu MC. The contribution of maternal stress to preterm birth: issues and considerations. *Clinical Perinatology*, 2011, 39:351–384.

13. Campbell JC. Health consequences of intimate partner violence. *The Lancet*, 2002, 359(9314):1331–1336.

14. Ellsberg M et al. Intimate partner violence and women's physical and mental health in the WHO multi-country study on women's health and domestic violence: an observational study. *The Lancet*, 2008, 371(9619):1165–1172.

15. García-Moreno C et al. Violence against women. *Science*, 2005, 310(5752):1282–1283.

16. Krug EG et al. The world report on violence and health. *The Lancet*, 2002, 360(9339):1083–1088.

17. Jansen HAFM et al. Interviewer training in the WHO multi-country study on women's health and domestic violence. *Violence Against Women,* 2004, 10(7):831–849.

18. Ellsberg M et al. Researching domestic violence against women: methodological and ethical considerations. *Studies in Family Planning*, 2001, 32(1):1–16.

19. University of New South Wales, Global Burden of Disease Mental Disorders and Illicit Drug Use Expert Group. *Regions* (http://www.gbd.unsw.edu.au/gbdweb.nsf/page/regions, accessed 8 April 2013).

20. Straus MA et al. The revised conflict tactics scales (CTS2). *Journal of Family Issues*, 1996, 17(3):283–316.

21. García-Moreno C et al. *WHO multi-country study on women's health and domestic violence against women: initial results on prevalence, health outcomes and women's responses*. Geneva, World Health Organization, 2005.

22. Kishor S, Johnson K. *Profiling domestic violence: a multi-country study*. Calverton, MD, MEASURE DHS+, ORC Macro, 2004.

23. Coker AL et al. Physical health consequences of physical and psychological intimate partner violence. *Archives of Family Medicine*, 2000, 9(5):451–457.

24. Jewkes R. Emotional abuse: a neglected dimension of partner violence. *The Lancet*, 2010, 376(9744):851–852.

25. Johnson H, Ollus, N, Nevala S. *Violence against women. An international perspective*. New York, Springer, 2008.

26. Hettige S. *GENACIS: gender, alcohol and culture: an international study* (http://genacis.org/, accessed 1 April 2013).

27. van Dijk JJM et al. *The burden of crime in the EU, a comparitive analysis of the European Survey of Crime and Safety* (EU ICS) 2005. Brussels, Gallup Europe, 2007.

28. Naudé CM, Prinsloo JH, Ladikos A. *Experiences of crime in thirteen African countries: results from the International Crime Victim Survey*, Turin, UNICRI-UNODC, 2006.

29. Peterman A, Palermo T, Bredenkamp C. Estimates and determinants of sexual violence against women in the Democratic Republic of Congo. *American Journal of Public Health*, 2011, 101(6):1060–1067.

30. Johnson K et al. Association of combatant status and sexual violence with health and mental health outcomes in post-conflict Liberia. *JAMA*, 2008, 300(6):676–690.

31. Johnson K et al., Association of sexual violence and human rights violations with physical and mental health in territories of the Eastern Democratic Republic of the Congo. *JAMA*, 2010, 304(5):553–562.

32. Hynes M et al. A determination of the prevalence of gender-based violence among conflict-affected populations in East Timor. *Disasters*, 2004, 28(3):294–321.

33. Swiss S et al. Violence against women during the Liberian civil conflict. *JAMA*, 1998, 279(8):625–629.

34. Amowitz LL et al. Prevalence of war-related sexual violence and other human rights abuses among internally displaced persons in Sierra Leone. *Journal of the American Medical Association*, 2002, 287(4):513–521.

35. StataCorp. *Intercooled Stata, Version 12.1. 11.0*. Houston: StataCorp, 2012.

36. Knapp G, Hartung J. Improved tests for a random effects meta-regression with a single covariate. *Statistics in Medicine*, 2003, 22:2693–2710.

37. Devries K et al. *Global prevalence of intimate partner violence against women* (draft manuscript; available upon request).

38. Abrahams N et al. *Global prevalence of non-partner sexual violence* (draft manuscript; available upon request).

39. United Nations. *Statistics and indicators on women and men* (http://unstats.un.org/unsd/demographic/products/indwm/default.htm, accessed 25 April 2013).

40. Secretariat of the Pacific Community. *Kiribati family health and safety study: a study on violence against women and children.* South Tarawa, Secretariat of the Pacific Community, 2010 (http://www.spc.int/hdp/index.php?option = com_docman&task = cat_view&gid = 89&Itemid = 44, accessed 8 April 2013).

41. Secretariat of the Pacific Community. *Solomon Islands Family Health and Safety Study: a study on violence against women and children.* Honiara, Secretariat of the Pacific Community, 2009 (http://www.spc.int/hdp/index.php?option = com_docman&task = cat_view&gid = 39&Itemid = 44, accessed 8 April 2013).

42. Vanuatu Women's Centre in Partnership with the Vanuatu National Statistics Office. *The Vanuatu National Survey on Women's Lives and Family Relationships.* Vanuatu, Vanuatu Women's Centre, 2011 (http://www.ausaid.gov.au/Publications/Pages/3407_3327_9971_6560_2865.aspx, accessed 8 April 2013).

43. Liberia Institute of Statistics and Geo-Information Services (LISGIS) (Liberia), Ministry of Health and Social Welfare (Liberia), National AIDS Control Program (Liberia), and Macro International Inc. *Liberia Demographic and Health Survey 2007.* Monrovia, Liberia Institute of Statistics and Geo-Information Services (LISGIS) and Macro International Inc., 2008 (http://www.measuredhs.com/pubs/pdf/FR201/FR201.pdf, accessed 10 April 2013).

44. García-Moreno C, Watts C. Violence against women: its importance for HIV/AIDS. *AIDS*, 2000, 14(Suppl. 3):S253–S265.

45. Maman S et al. The intersections of HIV and violence: directions for future research and interventions. *Social Science and Medicine*, 2000, 50(4):459–478.

46. Andersson N, Cockcroft A, Shea B. Gender-based violence and HIV: relevance for HIV prevention in hyperendemic countries of southern Africa. *AIDS*, 2008, 22(Suppl. 4):S73–S86.

47. Campbell JC et al. The intersection of intimate partner violence against women and HIV/AIDS: a review. *International Journal of Injury Control and Safety Promotion*, 2008, 15(4):221–231.

48. Coker AL. Does physical intimate partner violence affect sexual health? A systematic review. *Trauma Violence and Abuse*, 2007, 8(2):149–177.

49. Fernandez-Botran R et al. Correlations among inflammatory markers in plasma, saliva and oral mucosal transudate in post-menopausal women with past intimate partner violence. *Brain, Behavior, and Immunity*, 2011, 25(2):314–321.

50. Newton TL, et al. Markers of inflammation in midlife women with intimate partner violence histories. *Journal of Women's Health*, 2011, 20(12):1871–1880.

51. Wingood GM, DiClemente RJ. The effects of an abusive primary partner on the condom use and sexual negotiation practices of African-American women [see comments]. *American Journal of Public Health*, 1997, 87(6):1016–1018.

52. Dunkle KL et al. Perpetration of partner violence and HIV risk behaviour among young men in the rural Eastern Cape, South Africa. *AIDS*, 2006, 20(16):2107–2114.

53. Abrahams N et al. Sexual violence against intimate partners in Cape Town: prevalence and risk factors reported by men. *Bulletin of the World Health Organization* Bulletin, 2004, 82(5):330–337.

54. Gilbert L et al. Intimate partner violence and HIV risks: a longitudinal study of men on methadone. *Journal of Urban Health, 2007,* 84(5):667–680.

55. Raj A et al. Perpetration of intimate partner violence associated with sexual risk behaviors among young adult men. *American Journal of Public Health*, 2006, 96(10):1873–1878.

56. Santana MC et al. Masculine gender roles associated with increased sexual risk and intimate partner violence perpetration among young adult men. *Journal of Urban Health*, 2006, 83(4):575–585.

57. Devries K et al. *Is intimate partner violence a risk factor for HIV and STI infection in women? A systematic review and meta-analysis* (draft manuscript; available upon request).

58. Jewkes RK et al. Intimate partner violence, relationship power inequity, and incidence of HIV infection in young women in South Africa: a cohort study. *The Lancet,* 2010, 376(9734):41–48.

59. Weiss HA et al. Spousal sexual violence and poverty are risk factors for sexually transmitted infections in women: a longitudinal study of women in Goa, India. *Sexually Transmitted Infections*, 2008, 84(2):133–139.

60. Zablotska IB et al. Alcohol use, intimate partner violence, sexual coercion and HIV among women aged 15–24 in Rakai, Uganda. *AIDS and Behavior*, 2009, 13(2):225–233.

61. El-Bassel N et al. HIV and intimate partner violence among methadone-maintained women in New York City. *Social Science and Medicine*, 2005, 61(1):171–183.

62. Maman S et al. HIV-positive women report more lifetime partner violence: findings from a voluntary counseling and testing clinic in Dar es Salaam, Tanzania. A*merican Journal of Public Health*, 2002, 92(8):1331–1337.

63. Diaz-Olavarrieta C et al. The co-occurrence of intimate partner violence and syphilis among pregnant women in Bolivia. J*ournal of Women's Health*, 2009 18(12):2077–2086.

64. Moore AM, Frohwirth L, Miller E. Male reproductive control of women who have experienced intimate partner violence in the United States. *Social Science and Medicine*, 2010, 70(11):1737–1744.

65. Goodwin MM et al. Pregnancy intendedness and physical abuse around the time of pregnancy: findings from the pregnancy risk assessment monitoring system, 1996–1997. *Maternal and Child Health Journal*, 2000, 4(2):85–92.

66. Pallitto CC, Campbell JC, O'Campo P. Is intimate partner violence associated with unintended pregnancy? A review of the literature. *Trauma, Violence, and Abuse*, 2005, 6(3):217–235.

67. Silverman JG et al. Intimate partner violence and unwanted pregnancy, miscarriage, induced abortion, and stillbirth among a national sample of Bangladeshi women. BJOG: An International *Journal of Obstetrics and Gynaecology*, 2007, 114(10):1246–1252.

68. Singh S. *Abortion worldwide: a decade of uneven progress*. New York, Guttmacher Institute, 2009.

69. Sedgh G et al. Induced abortion: incidence and trends worldwide from 1995 to 2008. *The Lancet* 2012, 379 (9816):625–632.

70. Pallitto C et al. *Intimate partner violence and abortion: results of a meta-analysis* (draft manuscript; available upon request).

71. Hill A, Pallitto C, Garcia-Moreno C. *Intimate partner violence during pregnancy as a risk factor for low birth weight, preterm birth, and intrauterine growth restriction: a systematic review and meta-analysis* (draft manuscript; available upon request).

72. Devries K et al. *Intimate partner violence victimization and alcohol consumption in women: a systematic review and meta-analysis* (draft manuscript; available upon request).

73. Vos T et al. Measuring the impact of intimate partner violence on the health of women in Victoria, Australia. *Bulletin of the World Health Organization*, 2006, 84:739–744.

74. Hyde JS, Mezulis AH, Abramson LY. The ABCs of depression: integrating affective, biological, and cognitive models to explain the emergence of the gender difference in depression. *Psychological Review*, 2008, 115(2):291–313.

75. Khalifeh H, Dean K. Gender and violence against people with severe mental illness. *International Review of Psychiatry*, 2010, 22(5):535–546.

76. McPherson M, Delva J, Cranford JA. A longitudinal investigation of intimate partner violence among mothers with mental illness. *Psychiatric Services*, 2007, 58(5):675–680.

77. Bifulco A et al. Adult attachment style as mediator between childhood neglect/abuse and adult depression and anxiety. *Social Psychiatry and Psychiatric Epidemiology*, 2006, 41(10):796–805.

78. Doumas DM et al. Adult attachment as a risk factor for intimate partner violence: the "mispairing" of partners' attachment styles. *Journal of Interpersonal Violence*, 2008, 23(5):616–634.

79. Devries K et al. Intimate partner violence and incident depressive symptoms and suicide attempts: a systematic review of longitudinal studies. *PLoS Medicine*, 2013, 10(5):e1001439.

80. Ackard DM, Eisenberg ME, Neumark-Sztainer D. Long-term impact of adolescent dating violence on the behavioral and psychological health of male and female youth. *Journal of Pediatrics*, 2007, 151(5):476–481.

81. Chowdhary N, Patel V. The effect of spousal violence on women's health: findings from the Stree Arogya Shodh in Goa, India. *Journal of Postgraduate Medicine*, 2008, 54(4):306–312.

82. Roberts TA, Klein JD, Fisher S. Longitudinal effect of intimate partner abuse on high-risk behavior among adolescents. *Archives of Pediatrics and Adolescent Medicine*, 2003, 157:875–881.

83. Sheridan DJ, Nash KR. Acute injury patterns of intimate partner violence victims. *Trauma, Violence, and Abuse*, 2007, 8(3):281–289.

84. Tjaden P, Thoennes N. *Extent, nature, and consequences of intimate partner violence: findings from the National Violence against Women Survey*. Washington DC, National Institute of Justice, 2000.

85. Pallitto C, Petzold M, Garcia-Moreno C. *Intimate partner violence and physical injuries: synthesis of the global evidence* (draft manuscript; available upon request).

86. Hegarty K et al. Physical and social predictors of partner abuse in women attending general practice: a cross-sectional study. *British Journal of General Practice*, 2008, 58(552):484–487.

87. McCauley J et al. The battering syndrome – prevalence and clinical characteristics of domestic violence in primary-care internal medicine practices. *Annals of Internal Medicine*, 1995, 123(10), 737–746.

88. Rachana C et al. Prevalence and complications of physical violence during pregnancy. European *Journal of Obstetrics, Gynecology, and Reproductive Biology*, 2002, 103(1):26–29.

89. Stöckl H et al. The global prevalence of intimate partner homicide *The Lancet*. (forthcoming).

90. Kimerling R et al. The Veterans Health Administration and military sexual trauma. American *Journal of Public Health*, 2007, 97(12)2160–2166.

91. *Diagnostic and statistical manual of mental disorders*, 4th ed. Arlington, VA, American Psychiatric Association, 1994.

92. Hankin CS et al. Prevalence of depressive and alcohol abuse symptoms among women VA outpatients who report experiencing sexual assault while in the military. *Journal of Traumatic Stress*, 1999, 12(4):601–612.

93. Kohout FJ et al. Two shorter forms of the CES-D Depression Symptoms Index. *Journal of Aging and Health*, 1993,. 5(2):179–193.

94. Plichta SB, Falik M. Prevalence of violence and its implications for women's health. *Women's Health Issues*, 2001, 11(3):244–258.

95. Richman JA et al. Sexual harassment and generalized workplace abuse among university employees: prevalence and mental health correlates. *American Journal of Public Health*, 1999, 89(3):358–363.

96. McNair D, Lorr M, Droppleman L. *Manual for the Profile of Mood States (POMS)*. San Diego, CA, Educational and Industrial testing Services, 1971.

97. Nicolaidis C et al. Violence, mental health, and physical symptoms in an academic internal medicine practice. *Journal of General Internal Medicine*, 2004, 19:819–827.

98. Derogatis LR, Lazarus L. SCL-90-R, *Brief Symptom Inventory, and matching clinical rating scales. The use of psychological testing for treatment planning and outcome assessment*. Hillsdale, NJ, Lawrence Erlbaum Associates, 1994.

99. Rospenda KM et al. Chronicity of sexual harassment and generalized work-place abuse: effects on drinking outcomes. *Addiction*, 2000, 95(12):1805–1820.

100. Tschumper A et al. Sexual victimization in adolescent girls (age 15–20 years) enrolled in post-mandatory schools or professional training programmes in Switzerland. *Acta Paediatrica*, 1998, 87:212–217.

101. Musayón Oblitas FY, Caufield C. Workplace violence and drug use in women workers in a Peruvian Barrio. *International Nursing Review*, 2007, 54(4):339–345.

102. Selzer ML. The Michigan Alcoholism Screening Test: the quest for a new diagnostic instrument. *American Journal of Psychiatry*, 1971, 127:1653–1658.

103. Golding JM et al. Sexual assault history and use of health and mental health services. *American Journal of Community Psychology*, 1988, 16(5):625–644.

104. Coker AL et al. Physical and mental health effects of intimate partner violence for men and women. *American Journal of Preventive Medicine*, 24(4):260–268.

105. Kendall-Tackett KA, Inflammation, cardiovascular disease, and metabolic syndrome as sequelae of violence against women – the role of depression, hostility and sleep disturbance. *Trauma, Violence, and Abuse*, 2007, 8(2):117–126.

106. Jejeebhoy SJ. Associations between wife-beating and fetal and infant death: impressions from a survey in rural India. *Studies in Family Planning*, 1998, 29(3):300–308.

107. Ziaei S, Naved RT, Ekström EC. Women's exposure to intimate partner violence and child malnutrition: findings from demographic and health surveys in Bangladesh. *Maternal and Child Nutrition*, 2012, Aug 20 doi: 10.1111/j.1740-8709.2012.00432.x.

108. Asling-Monemi K, Naved RT, Persson LA. Violence against women and increases in the risk of diarrheal disease and respiratory tract infections in infancy: a prospective cohort study in Bangladesh. *Archives of Pediatrics and Adolescent Medicine*, 2009, 163(10):931–936.

109. Asling-Monemi K, Naved RT, Persson LA. Violence against women and the risk of fetal and early childhood growth impairment: a cohort study in rural Bangladesh. *Archives of Disease in Childhood*, 2009, 94(10):775–779.

110. World Health Organization. *Responding to intimate partner violence and sexual violence against women: WHO clinical and policy guidelines.* Geneva, World Health Organization, 2013.

111. World Health Organization. *Preventing intimate partner violence and sexual violence against women. Taking action and generating evidence.* Geneva, World Health Organization, 2010.

112. Heise L. *What works to prevent partner violence? An evidence overview.* London: Crown Copyright, 2011 (https://www.gov.uk/government/news/dfid-research-what-works-to-prevent-violence-against-women-by-their-partners, accessed 1 April 2013).

113. Jewkes R, Nduna M, Jama Shai N, Dunkle K. *Prospective study of rape perpetration by young South African men: incidence & risk factors.* PLoS One. 2012;7(5):e38210.

114. Naved R T, Huque H, et al. (2011). *Men's attitudes and practices regarding gender and violence against women in Bangladesh.* Preliminary findings. Dhaka, ICDDR,B.

115. The World Bank. *Country and lending groups* (http://data.worldbank.org/about/country-classifications/country-and-lending-groups, accessed 10 April 2013).

Appendix 1: Countries included by WHO region and age group

Table A1.1. Countries included in intimate partner violence prevalence estimates by WHO region

WHO region	Countries
Low- and middle-income regions:	
Africa	Botswana, Cameroon, Democratic Republic of the Congo, Ethiopia, Kenya, Lesotho, Liberia, Malawi, Mozambique, Namibia, Rwanda, South Africa, Swaziland, Uganda, United Republic of Tanzania, Zambia, Zimbabwe
Americas	Brazil, Chile, Colombia, Costa Rica, Dominican Republic, Ecuador, El Salvador, Haiti, Honduras, Jamaica, Mexico, Nicaragua, Paraguay, Peru, Plurinational State of Bolivia
Eastern Mediterranean	Egypt, Iran, Iraq, Jordan, Palestine[a]
Europe	Albania, Azerbaijan, Georgia, Lithuania, Republic of Moldova, Romania, Russian Federation, Serbia, Turkey, Ukraine
South-East Asia	Bangladesh, Timor-Leste (East Timor), India, Myanmar, Sri Lanka, Thailand
Western Pacific	Cambodia, China, Philippines, Samoa, Viet Nam
High income[b]	Australia, Canada, Croatia, Czech Republic, Denmark, Finland, France, Germany, Hong Kong,[a] Iceland, Ireland, Israel, Japan, Netherlands, New Zealand, Norway, Poland, South Korea, Spain, Sweden, Switzerland, United Kingdom of Great Britain and Northern Ireland, United States of America

[a] Data from this territory (not a WHO Member State) were included in the regional estimates.

[b] High-income countries are classified by the World Bank based on the gross national income per capita calculated using the World Bank Atlas method (*115*).

Table A1.2. Countries included in non-partner sexual violence prevalence estimates by WHO region

WHO region	Countries
Low- and middle-income regions:	
Africa	Burkina Faso, Democratic Republic of the Congo, Ethiopia, Ghana, Kenya, Liberia, Malawi, Mozambique, Namibia, Nigeria, Sierra Leone, South Africa, Uganda, United Republic of Tanzania, Zambia, Zimbabwe
Americas	Argentina, Belize, Brazil, Costa Rica, Jamaica, Nicaragua, Peru, Uruguay
Eastern Mediterranean	
Europe	Azerbaijan, Kazakhstan, Kosovo, Lithuania, Serbia, Turkey, Ukraine
South-East Asia	Bangladesh, Timor-Leste (East Timor), India, Maldives, Sri Lanka, Thailand
Western Pacific	Kiribati, Philippines, Samoa
High income[a]	Australia, Canada, Czech Republic, Denmark, Finland, Germany, Hong Kong,[b] Isle of Man,[b] Japan, New Zealand, Poland, Spain, Sweden, Switzerland, United Kingdom of Great Britain and Northern Ireland, United States of America

[a] High-income countries are classified by the World Bank based on the gross national income per capita calculated using the World Bank Atlas method (*115*).

[b] Data from this territory (not a WHO Member State) were included in the regional estimates.

Table A1.3. **Number of estimates included in analysis of intimate partner violence by WHO region and age group**

Age group, years	Low and middle-income regions						High income	Total
	Africa	Americas	Eastern Mediterranean	Europe	Western Pacific	South-East Asia		
15–19	44	60	9	29	12	16	28	198
20–24	44	59	7	15	20	16	38	199
25–29	42	59	8	29	18	16	34	206
30–34	44	60	9	31	20	16	36	216
35–39	5	18	2	8	11	1	28	73
40–44	2	13	2	6	6	1	4	34
45–49	42	59	7	10	26	16	31	191
50–54	0	4	1	0	6	0	2	13
55–59	0	4	0	0	0	0	3	13
60–64	2	0	0	0	0	0	5	7
65–69	3	3	1	0	3	0	23	33

Table A1.4. **Number of estimates included in analysis of intimate partner violence by region for all ages combined**

Age group	Low and middle-income regions						High income	Total
	Africa	Americas	Eastern Mediterranean	Europe	Western Pacific	South-East Asia		
All ages combined	71	72	18	50	33	34	114	392

Appendix 2: Prevalence estimates of violence against women by Global Burden of Disease regions

Intimate partner violence

When the prevalence data are grouped by the 21 regions used in the 2010 Global Burden of Disease (GBD) study, a more nuanced picture appears. The highest prevalence is found in central sub-Saharan Africa, where a prevalence of 65.6% of ever-partnered women have experienced intimate partner violence. All regions of sub-Saharan Africa are above the global average of 26.4%. The lowest prevalence is in East Asia, with 16.3% of ever-partnered women reporting intimate partner violence. The only other regions below the global average are high-income Western Europe (19.3%), North America (21.3%), Central Asia (22.9%) and Southern Latin America (23.7%). The remaining countries have a prevalence of 26% or above. It is important to note that even in the case of the below-average regions, between one quarter and one fifth of ever-partnered women have still experienced partner violence.

Table A.2.1. Prevalence of intimate partner violence by GBD region

Region	Prevalence (95% confidence interval), %
Asia Pacific, High Income	28.45 (20.6 to 36.3)
Asia, Central	22.89 (15.8 to 30.0)
Asia, East	16.30 (8.9 to 23.7)
Asia, South	41.73 (36.3 to 47.2)
Asia, South-East	27.99 (23.7 to 32.2)
Australasia	28.29 (22.7 to 33.9)
Caribbean	27.09 (20.8 to 33.3)
Europe, Central	27.85 (22.7 to 33.0)
Europe, Eastern	26.13 (20.6 to 31.6)
Europe, Western	19.30 (15.9 to 22.7)
Latin America, Andean	40.63 (34.8 to 46.5)
Latin America, Central	29.51 (24.6 to 34.4)
Latin America, Southern	23.68 (12.8 to 34.5)
Latin America, Tropical	27.43 (20.7 to 34.2)
North Africa/Middle East	35.38 (30.4 to 40.3)
North America, High Income	21.32 (16.2 to 26.4)
Oceania	35.27 (23.8 to 46.7)
Sub-Saharan Africa, Central	65.64 (53.6 to 77.7)
Sub-Saharan Africa, East	38.83 (34.6 to 43.1)
Sub-Saharan Africa, Southern	29.67 (24.3 to 35.1)
Sub-Saharan Africa, West	41.75 (32.9 to 50.6)

Non-partner sexual violence

This section presents additional data on the prevalence estimates of non-partner sexual violence, grouped by the 21 regions from the GBD 2010 study. There were variations across the regions, with the prevalence ranging between 3.3% and 21.0%. The highest prevalence was reported in the sub-Saharan Africa, Central region (21%) followed by the sub-Saharan Africa Southern (17.4%) region. The large confidence interval in the sub-Saharan Africa, Central region is most likely due to this being based on a single estimate. The lowest estimate was reported in the Asia South region (3.3 %), followed by the North Africa/Middle East region (4.5%).

Table A.2.2. Prevalence of non-partner sexual violence by GBD region

Region	Prevalence (95% confidence interval), %
Asia Pacific, High Income	12.20 (4.21 to 20.19)
Asia, Central	6.45 (0 to 13.0)
Asia, East	5.87 (0.15 to 11.59)
Asia, South	3.35 (0 to 8.37)
Asia, South-East	5.28 (0.94 to 9.61)
Australasia	16.46 (11.52 to 21.41)
Caribbean	10.32 (3.71 to 16.92)
Europe, Central	10.76 (6.14 to 15.38)
Europe, Eastern	6.97 (0 to 14.13)
Europe, Western	11.50 (7.24 to 15.76)
Latin America, Andean	15.33 (10.12 to 20.54)
Latin America, Central	11.88 (7.31 to 16.45)
Latin America, Southern	5.86 (0.31 to 11.42)
Latin America, Tropical	7.68 (2.68 to 12.69)
North Africa/Middle East	4.53 (0 to 12.74)
North America, High Income	13.01 (9.02 to 16.99)
Oceania	14.86 (7.48 to 22.24)
Sub-Saharan Africa, Central	21.05 (4.59 to 37.51)
Sub-Saharan Africa, East	11.46 (7.31 to 15.60)
Sub-Saharan Africa, Southern	17.41 (11.48 to 23.33)
Sub-Saharan Africa, West	9.15 (4.90 to 13.41)

Appendix 3: Regression models for calculating regional estimates of intimate partner violence

Regression function to estimate regional levels of intimate partner violence

Intercept is omitted in the model:

$$\text{Prevalence}_i = \beta_1 * \text{subnational} + \beta_2 * \text{physvio} + \beta_3 * \text{sexvio} + \beta_4 * \text{pastyr} + \beta_5 * \text{severity} + \beta_6 * \text{notviostudy} + \beta_7 * \text{nointrain} + \beta_8 * \text{pstatus} + \beta_9 * \text{region}_1 + \ldots + \beta_{15} * \text{region}_7 + \mu_i$$

where μ_i is the residual for the i:th study estimate, and the dummy variables are coded as:

- subnational = 0 if national, 1 if subnational;
- physvio = 0 if physical and/or sexual intimate partner violence, 1 if physical violence only;
- sexvio = 0 if physical and/or sexual intimate partner violence, 1 if sexual violence only;
- pastyr = 0 if lifetime exposure to intimate partner violence, 1 if past-year violence only;
- severity = 0 if any form of intimate partner violence, 1 if severe violence only;
- notviostudy = 0 if study designed to measure violence, 1 if study not indented to measure violence;
- nointrain = 0 if interviewers trained, 1 if not trained;
- pstatus = 0 if ever-partnered women included, 1 if only currently partnered women included;
- region_1 to region_7 are coded as 1 if study from corresponding region, 0 otherwise.

Regression function to estimate age-group-specific regional levels of intimate partner violence

Intercept is omitted in the model:

$$\text{Prevalence}_i = \beta_1 * \text{subnational} + \beta_2 * \text{physvio} + \beta_3 * \text{sexvio} + \beta_4 * \text{pastyr} + \beta_5 * \text{severity} + \beta_6 * \text{notviostudy} + \beta_7 * \text{nointrain} + \beta_8 * \text{pstatus} + \beta_{jk} * \text{region}_j * \text{agegroup}_k + \mu_i$$

where $\text{region}_j * \text{agegroup}_k$ denotes all main effects and interactions for all the combinations of regions and age groups, μ_i is the residual for the i:th study estimate, and the dummy variables are coded above.

Regression function to estimate regional levels for non-partner sexual violence

Intercept is omitted in the model:

$$\text{Prevalence}_i = \beta_1 * \text{subnational} + \beta_2 * \text{nointrain} + \beta_3 * \text{allnonpartners} + \beta_4 * \text{region}_1 + \ldots + \beta_{11} * \text{region}_7 + \mu_i$$

where μ_i is the residual for the i:th study estimate, and the dummy variables are coded as:

- subnational = 0 if national, 1 if subnational;
- nointrain = 0 if interviewers trained, 1 if not trained;
- allnonpartners = 0 if not all nonpartners included, 1 if all nonpartners included;
- region$_1$ to region$_7$ are coded as 1 if study from corresponding region, 0 otherwise.